# *A Cosmetic Surgery Recovery Guide*

**Christopher Saunders, MD, FACS, PA**

# Introduction:

Cosmetic surgery can provide wonderful and fantastic improvements to many people. The operations can make us look younger, thinner, flatter, and more healthy. They are extremely reliable, safe, and effective. But cosmetic surgery is *real* surgery which means that we have to proceed wisely and carefully. It is important to understand all aspects of your cosmetic surgery including the surgeon, technical aspects, expectations, and also the recovery.

Patients are often extremely happy after they wake up from their cosmetic operation. This is normal and natural. However the operation may be finished, but we still have to navigate the recovery process to get to the finish line safely. We must learn about recovery and what to do to maximize our chances of success and to have the least risk of problems. In my book the focus is to provide the reader with a complete cosmetic surgery recovery guide. The book emphasizes recovering from your procedures in the wisest and safest manner. Sometimes after surgery people forget or don't understand how important the recovery process is to assure the best results and safest healing. If this happens, patients can get worse results or the development of problems that could otherwise have been avoided by focusing on recovery. *Recovery is a critical part of all cosmetic surgery operations.*

This is my third book on cosmetic surgery. The first book was titled **A Woman's Guide to the "Real- Reality" of Cosmetic Surgery.** My second book was titled **A Tricky Fountain of Youth - Understanding Cosmetic Surgery.** The first two books focused on understanding critical concepts and realistic expectations about cosmetic surgery. I believe that understanding expectations and what cosmetic surgery can really achieve is of paramount importance. These books are excellent reference sources, and I encourage the interested person to read them.

I have been practicing plastic surgery for over 25 years and perform exclusively cosmetic surgery. I have performed over 50,000 cosmetic surgery operations and procedures. During my career, I have been lucky to receive more awards than I can count from my peers and patients on cosmetic and plastic surgery. I have many national and international publications and presentations on cosmetic and plastic surgery. These have been the fruit of studying and working extremely hard over my entire medical career. I strive to provide the highest quality cosmetic surgery care that I think is possible. I spent much time and effort working on this book to help patients and readers understand and learn about the best way to recover from cosmetic surgery. I hope you find the book valuable and interesting.

**Note to Reader:**

This book is designed to be a guide and a source of information to the reader. It will help a person considering cosmetic surgery be more informed and educated about recovering from cosmetic surgery. It is impossible to be a complete reference source and additional information should be found when necessary and appropriate. Additional information on cosmetic surgery can be found on my webpage **ChrisSaundersMD.com.**

I am an expert in the field of cosmetic surgery. This book represents my extensive experience and opinions. It is not meant to be the only resource and other sources may be helpful to you as a patient. The book may not reflect everyone's position. There are differences in opinion, and other doctors might not agree with a given topic or information. In this book, I discuss concepts and information in an educational format. You should contact your doctor to determine if a given procedure can be of benefit to you.

Before undergoing any cosmetic procedure or operation it is essential to have an in-depth consultation with a board-certified plastic surgeon. You must have a thorough discussion of any and all risks, benefits, and options. This book can help you be more educated and informed about this important decision. Cosmetic surgery procedures are usually extremely safe and effective in the majority of patients. However, no operation is without risk. It is important that all patients considering cosmetic surgery and reading this book have a complete and thorough understanding of the surgery, risks, and recovery.

**Acknowledgments:**

Writing a cosmetic surgery book and having a surgical career take an extremely large amount of time away from your family and loved ones. This book is dedicated to my family. I love them very much!

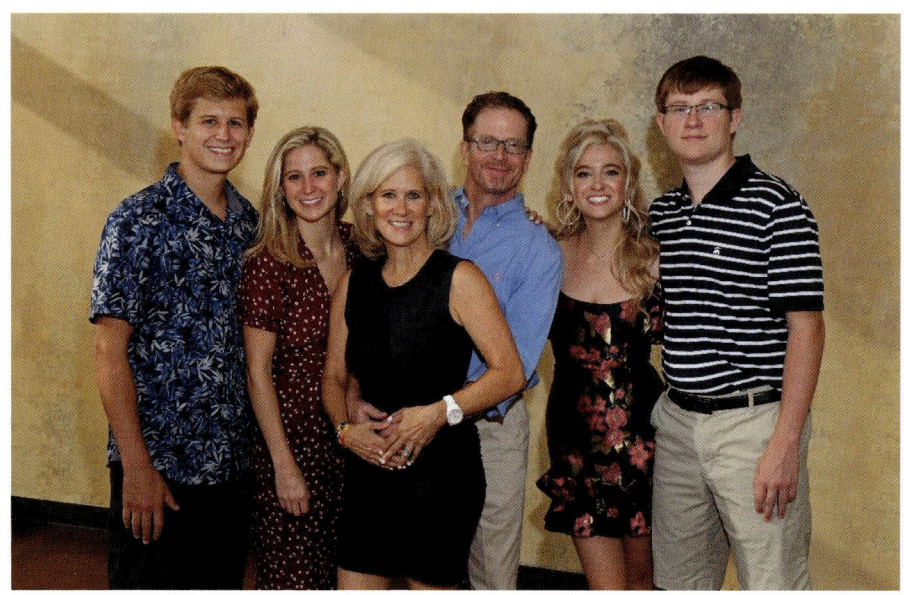

A recent family photograph.

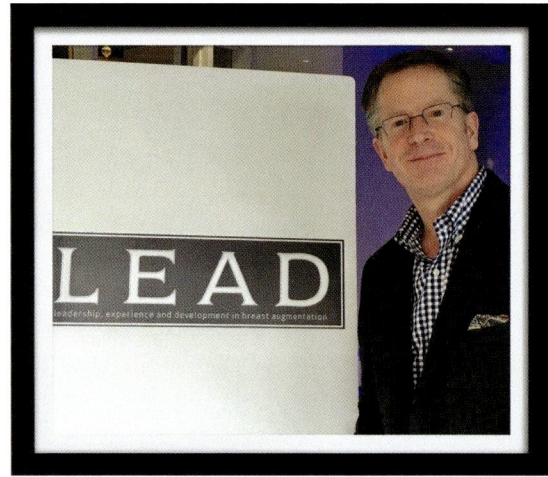
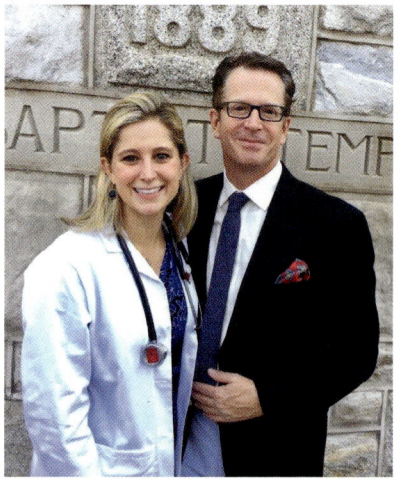

A photograph of me after presenting at a recent meeting and
the fourth generation doctor, Lexi Saunders, at Temple medical school.

# Table of Contents

Chapter 1

# Recovering from Cosmetic Surgery

Cosmetic surgery can be a fountain of youth for many people. The surgery can help you look younger, thinner, and more healthy. Success and satisfaction rates are usually extremely high for most cosmetic procedures. The decision to proceed with cosmetic surgery should be viewed as one of the most important decisions that you will make. This decision should be well thought out and planned. It should include carefully picking your surgeon, studying surgical techniques and methods, and reviewing results and photographs. However, once the operation is done, recovering from the procedure is just as important as the decision to do it. The recovery is just as critical as the preparation before surgery and the surgery itself. To maximize our chance of the best results, patients must understand that the recovery is an essential part of the entire cosmetic operation.

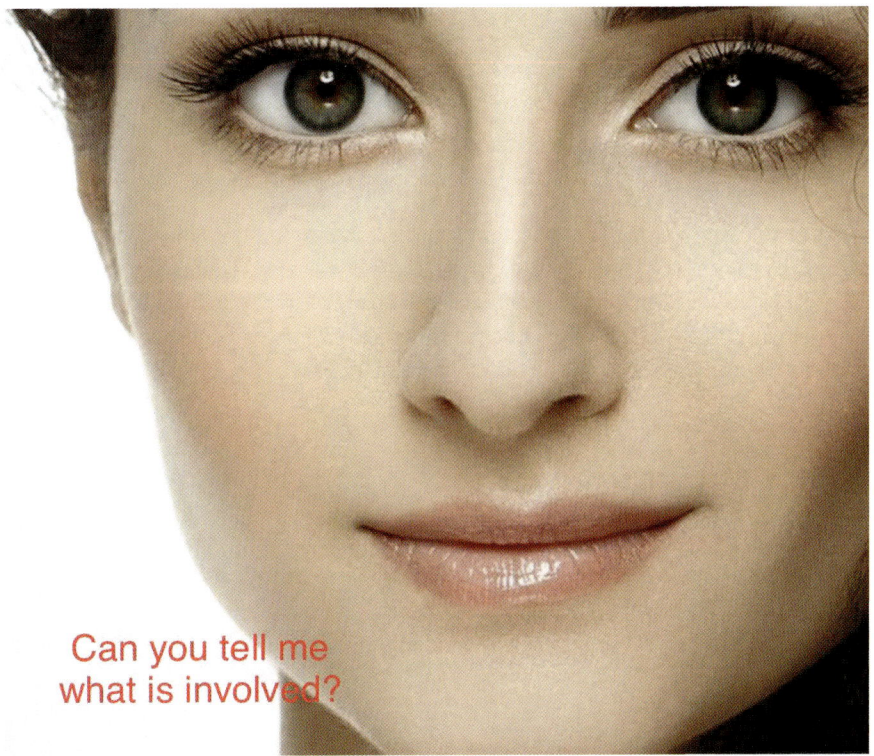

Can you tell me
what is involved?

The American Society of Plastic Surgery records the total number of major operations and procedures performed by plastic surgeons each year. Last year there were over 1.8 million major operations done in the USA and over 15 million minor procedures! Extensive study and review of these results show high success and satisfaction rates. This is one of the reasons so many people are interested and proceed with these procedures. However, in my opinion, there is an under emphasis on the importance of the recovery process. It's not just plastic surgery or cosmetic surgery, but recovery is not emphasized in many fields of medicine. This includes recovery from lacerations, burns, trauma, cancers, infections, orthopedics, and almost all operative fields.

After surgery the body goes through a complicated and intricate biochemical healing process. The sequence of healing goes through a series of stages. This includes inflammation followed by epithelization. Subsequently, the healing body goes through the processes of contraction and collagen synthesis. These are a complicated and interwoven series of physiologic steps that finishes with successful healing. During this healing process, if a patient does not follow the recommended steps, things could become interrupted with an increased chance of complications. It is obvious to most; we do not want to disrupt anything and adversely affect our chances of having the best results.

**Simple yet Strict:**

This book is being written to help patients learn about the recovery process and how to heal the best after cosmetic surgery. All the recovery instructions outlined will be straightforward or simple. The instructions are not going to be complex mathematical equations that are difficult to follow. The instructions will be clearly outlined and will be easy to follow. I phrase this as "simple yet strict." The instructions are not complicated, but they must be followed in every detail! Small changes in the instructions could lead to increased risks or problems. It's not complicated. The instructions are "simple yet strict."

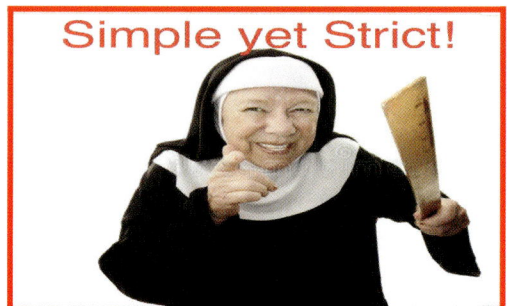

**Overall Concepts of Recovery:**

It is my job as a surgeon to teach you what is necessary to be done during recovery. I provide extensive information that is given to you following a cosmetic procedure. The information is also available on my webpage ChrisSaundersMD.com. All patients receive my personal cell phone, so they can contact me with questions or concerns regarding their surgery and recovery. I believe there are two critical components of recovery. These are understanding the "team approach" and the concept of "be the turtle." These are described in the following sections.

**Team Approach:**

It is your responsibility as a patient to listen intently to all instructions given. It is also important to review resources given on my webpage to help with learning and understanding about your operation and the recovery. It is vital to understand that recovery is also a team approach. You can't do it alone! Many things in medicine are team approaches. This means it's not just a doctor and the patient, but also family, nurses, and any other support staff that are helping you heal and recover. We obviously aren't going to be able to heal well if we're running around after the family dog or children after surgery. This could lead to increased risks and problems related to healing. The entire team must understand the importance of the surgery, the instructions, and everything that must be done to cross the finish line successfully.

**Be the Turtle:**

This is one of my favorite expressions when describing recovery. "Be the turtle" is another way of saying slow and steady wins the race. In the old fable about the tortoise and the hare, the hare (or rabbit) rushes ahead trying to get to the finish line the fastest. He always loses the race to the turtle who proceeds slowly and safely. You cannot rush healing or recovery. You cannot rush the important physiologic changes that are occurring to our body during

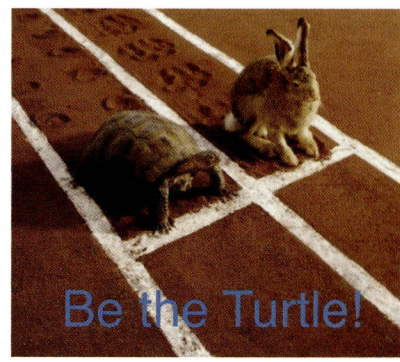

the healing process. If you do rush, you lead to increased chances of complications or risks. I believe it is impossible to over emphasize the importance of going slow and steady. When I say "be the turtle" it means - let's win this race. It means let's go slow. So we can all be happy after a successful cosmetic surgery operation.

After surgery you will be given specific and important tasks and instructions to help you heal. In the paragraphs above, I have reviewed general and overall concepts that are important to the best healing. What follows below are instructions for you that apply to all cosmetic procedures. It is an overview of things that you should focus on as you are preparing and recovering from your surgery.

## 1: Learn

Learn about your operation and what is involved to heal. This includes not just the consultation with the doctor but information that is available on his webpage and/or other medical sites. I recommend ChrisSaundersMD.com for my surgeries. But PlasticSurgery.org is the webpage of the American Society of Plastic Surgery. It is an excellent source of reference as well. Be careful about going to random web pages or blogs. These sites can skew the medical information and actually have information that is incorrect, not completely true, or unhelpful. In general, it is best to stick with your doctors' information or the PlasticSurgery.org.

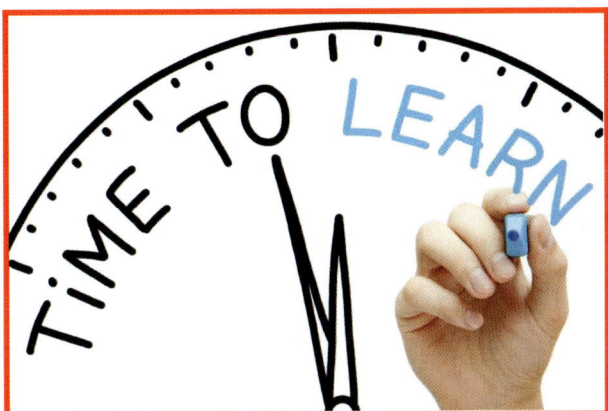

Read all the information that is provided. Read the information before surgery, during the recovery, and probably a third and fourth time. I have educational writings on my web page that I recommend my patients read. In the early postoperative period after surgery, I encourage them to read it again. They will gather information and learn material that might not have seemed important the first time they read it. You cannot learn too much about recovery from your operation.

## 2: Prepare

Prepare for your surgery. In addition to the learning process described above, this means getting everything ready and prepared so you have no problems after surgery. This means getting the team, as described above under team approach, prepared. Make sure people who are taking care of you after surgery have an appropriate amount of time off of work. Make sure people that you are responsible for children or animals have appropriate time to set up. Sometimes dogs need to be placed in a kennel, as larger dogs can't be walked easily after an operation.

If you are instructed to purchase anything such as compression garments, ice packs, or leg compression stockings, be prepared and have these purchased before surgery. I give all my patients their postoperative medication prescriptions before surgery, so they can be prepared and have them on the day of surgery. In this way they don't

have to run to the pharmacy after their operation but have everything ready and waiting. Remember the old adage - an ounce of preparation is worth a pound of cure. Be wise and be prepared for your operation.

## 3: Follow Through

Follow through with all your instructions. They are not always easy. Some people feel that they have the right to just follow the instructions that they want to. Others will do it their way and tell me, "This is the way I do it." I want you to do it the way I have instructed you to do it. Follow through with recovery instructions specifically. Most of these operations I've done a 1000 times or more. You, as an individual patient, have probably limited experience, so following the doctors' way is wise. Follow the instructions specifically. The reason you have them is because experience has shown patients will heal better and get better results.

## 4: Ask Questions

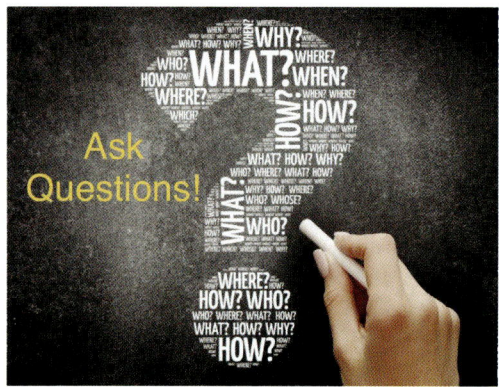

Ask questions at any time. As I have said, all patients will have my cell phone. If something is not understood, ask questions for a better or more thorough explanation. Ask for additional information if it is needed or desired. It is always important to ask questions. I tell my patients during the recovery process that all follow up visits will be in a specific order : patient examination followed by instructions followed by patient questions. Patient questions might come last, but the questions are probably the most important of all.

## 5: Change

Be prepared for postoperative instructions to change. Activity instructions will change. Initially after some operations, activity will be limited to minimize risk of injury to the muscle work or the delicate incisions. Activity will gradually increase and this will be one of the instructions given to you, but other instructions will change as well. Some patients will erroneously think that they were given the instructions already and so they know the answer over the next several months. But instructions change as you heal. They are modified and changed to be appropriate for the stage of your recovery. It is important to come to your follow up visits as instructions might change over time.

## Summary

After having cosmetic surgery, it is important to remember that the recovery process is part of the overall healing. Do not take the recovery process lightly. Is important to learn everything and to be prepared for what you are instructed to do. Follow through with these instructions, ask questions, and be prepared for the answers to change as you heal. Don't forget that recovery is a team approach, and it is important to "be the turtle" and to go slow and steady during the healing. The rest of the book will outline specific operations in cosmetic surgery that I perform. It will outline important recovery tasks and concepts that will give us the best chance of healing uneventfully.

Chapter 2

# General Post Operative Instructions

This chapter focuses on instructions that are important for all cosmetic or plastic surgery operations. Think of it as a general instruction sheet to recover from your operation. Additional and more specific instructions related to cosmetic operations can be found in the specific chapter for that operation. Patients should read this general instruction chapter but also the specific chapter for the operation they are doing. All postoperative instructions are meant to be as thorough and as complete as possible. However, there will always be the possibility of additional questions or concerns. Patients should not hesitate to call me for any problems.

In addition to specific instructions provided, it is important to remember that there are things you should not do! I call this the *do not do list.* This topic of the do not do list is covered in detail in chapter 3. It will review things that are prohibited and not allowed. This includes, but is not limited to, smoking, hot tubs, bathing, heating pads, and heavy lifting. This chapter is mandatory reading for all patients.

Another general and important concept after surgery is to "Be Wise." No matter how thorough or complete the instructions, there is always the possibility of a point being missed, misunderstood, or not emphasized. As a patient, remember to go slow and take your time. Think about what you are doing and why. Ask questions. Remember, it might sound like a cliche, but "Be Wise" during recovery after surgery, so we can heal safely.

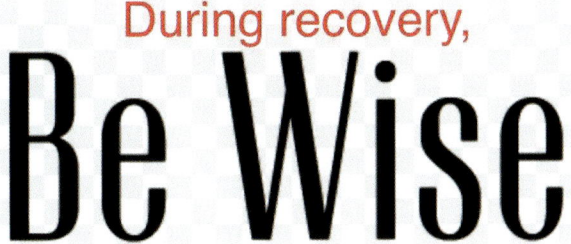

**General Instructions**:

Call me for:
1: Fevers over 101.5 degrees
2: Excessive bleeding
3: Excessive pain
4: Problems or concerns

After surgery it is extremely important to follow instructions closely. Not doing this can lead to increased complications and/or risks. These instructions are for one month from the date of your surgery. This may change and will be dependent on me clearing you for activities after surgery. Follow up visits are very important.

**Smoking:**

Smoking is probably the absolute worst thing you can do around surgery. It can lead to increased complications, scarring, and even loss or necrosis of tissue. I review this topic in depth in Chapter 4.

**Diet:**

After surgery patients should slowly advance their diet to normal as tolerated. Begin with liquids and light foods before progressing to a normal diet. You should start with clear liquids, crackers, banana or yogurt. Advancing a diet too quickly can lead to nausea and vomiting and hinder recovery. Remember, it is also good to have food in your stomach when taking medications. This helps decrease nausea and vomiting that can be associated with certain medications, such as pain medications.

**Medications:**

All of my patients are typically prescribed four medications. This includes an antibiotic, pain, nausea, and anxiety medications. The antibiotic is meant to be started when you go home. All patients receive intravenous antibiotics preoperatively. This is prophylactic to minimize the risk of infection. The course of oral antibiotics starts when you get home. The pain pills, anxiety pills, and nausea pills are considered PRN. This means that they are "as necessary" medications and are taken when and only if needed.

I usually prescribe Valium as an anxiety medicine. It is important to know that this medication also is an antispasmodic which can help with pain associated with some surgical procedures. Tummy tucks have muscle repair and can have pain associated with muscle spasm. The Valium can help with this pain, in addition to the pain medication prescribed. The nausea medicine and the pain medication should be taken as prescribed on the bottles. It is safe to add Advil or Tylenol to help with additional pain if encountered or needed. The maximum dose of Advil, Motrin, or ibuprofen is 12 tablets in a given day. 4 tablets taken at a time (800 mg) can give better pain relief than just taking two tablets.

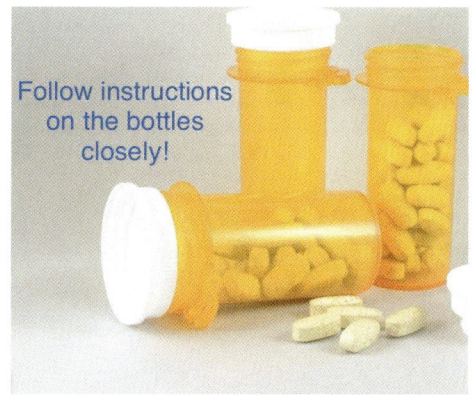

Follow instructions on the bottles closely!

**Bandages and Dressings:**

It is normal to have bloody drainage after surgery. This is typical and in general the first bandage will be slightly bloody. Don't be frightened as this is common. It is typically changed the morning after surgery during an office visit. If you feel that it is too bloody, the bandage can be reinforced with additional gauze, until your visit the next day in the office. If you decide to reinforce the bandage, please wash your hands thoroughly and do not touch the incision or drainage tubes where they exit from the skin.

**Incisions and Scars:**

Please see scar care and treatment in chapter 6. The entire chapter is devoted to this topic.

## Garments:

You will be provided with a compression garment or binder that is placed on you after surgery. They should be worn as much as possible for approximately 6 weeks. You can be out of the garment for a short period of time to wash and dry it. If the surgery is performed in the hot summer months, it can be taken off for comfort and reapplied when you are in a cooler or air-conditioned location.

Some people will choose to buy or obtain a second garment. The concept is pressure where you had surgery. So the garment can be any color or fabric, it just needs to be moderately tight. The pressure should not be too loose, and it should not be too tight, but a more medium tightness.

A second garment is nice as it allows for washing of the first one when the second one is being worn. Many garments are crotch-less to allow for easy urination without having to take the garments off. But this is an option, and it is not a required aspect of the garment. Spanx and Flexees are common brands of compression garments that I like.

## Showering:

Usually showering is allowed 72 hours or 3 days after surgery. Notice how I say showers are ok. But hot tubs or bathing is strictly forbidden!  This is typically for 6 weeks.

It is common to feel lightheaded at the first shower, and it is recommended to have someone help you with the shower. You should also have a sitting stool. If you feel lightheaded, please sit down and rest. It will usually pass in 5 to 10 minutes, and you'll feel normal again. After the shower, no gauze is necessary for the incision, as it has sealed.

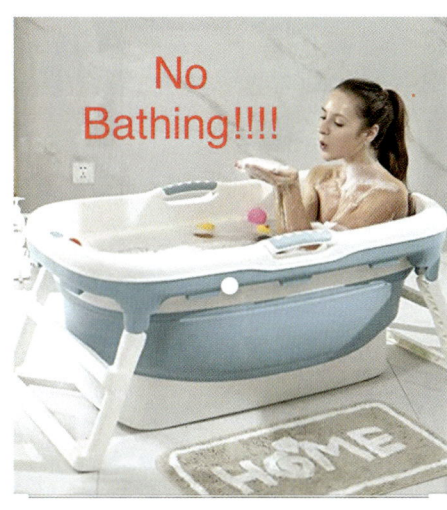

## Heat application:

No heat application to any surgical site or surrounding area. This can burn the skin severely. This includes heating pads, electric blankets, or hot water bottles. The skin can be numb after surgery and the feeling that things are too hot can be affected. The heat can lead to major injury and is absolutely forbidden.

## Activities:

Rest and relaxation are important after most operations. Too much activity after surgery or too little activity can be problematic. In general it is important to be "up and about" after surgery. Too little activity while in bed or on the couch after surgery, can lead to blood clots. This is why early ambulation after surgery is recommended. This usually means out of bed for 5 to 10 minutes 5 to 10 times a day. Conversely, too much activity can hinder healing and lead to increased bruising and bleeding. Activities such as shopping, cooking, laundry, and cleaning should be avoided until approved by me. It is imperative to read the chapter on blood clot prevention. In my opinion, this is one of the most important recovery instructions for all patients having any surgery! Please see Chapter 5.

After most cosmetic surgery operations, you will be instructed on your activity. It is important to understand that this will change from just after surgery to when you have healed and have unlimited exercise or activity. From the very beginning, it is important to get up out of bed and move around to minimize blood clots. This has been emphasized in multiple locations in this book. For the first week, patients should as a minimum get out of bed 5 to 10 times a day for approximately 5 to 10 minutes.

After this first week, activity can slowly and gradually increase. I called it a "phased-in" recovery. What this means is during the first week we might predominantly be at home and just walking around the house. We are moving our legs and ambulating to minimize the risk of blood clots, but not overdoing it and potentially increasing risks or problems. After approximately 1 or 2 weeks, until 6 weeks, we have gradually increased or "phased-in" recovery. During this period activity is slowly increased.

This "phased-in" recovery means that stationary bicycles, ellipticals, or walking on a treadmill are acceptable when approved by me after about 2 weeks. But running, weightlifting, CrossFit, or more strenuous exercise is not allowed. At the end of 6 weeks, if you are doing well, most people can resume all exercise and/or activity including heavy lifting. The specific length of time that you will be restricted depends on each individual operation. In general the guiding concept is that initially we are taking it easy, and then we slowly phase in our exercise and activity to a period when we have no limitations.

**Restrictions:**

Please do not use heating pads, electric blankets, or hot water bottles to any surgical site. Refrain from sexual activity until further notice. No smoking has been emphasized.
Please see Chapter 3 on the "Do Not Do" list.

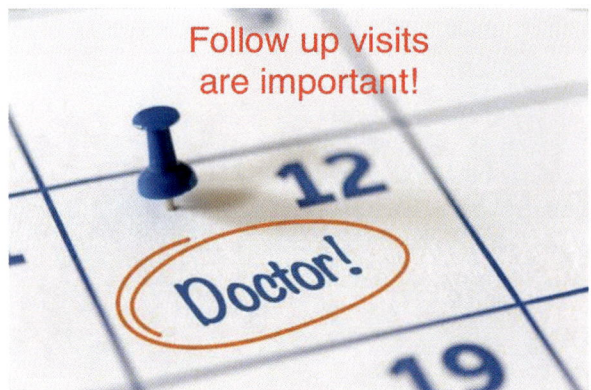

**Follow up care:**

I see most patients the day after surgery for a postoperative check. Liposuction and rhinoplasty patients might be seen 2 or 3 days after surgery depending on the day of the week surgery is performed. Office visits are extremely important because they allow me to make sure everything is healing well. Also, in the unlikely event of something going wrong, I can pick it up earlier. Earlier treatments can mean better results and outcomes. Even follow up visits that seem long after surgery are important. Instructions will change as you heal. Keep coming to your visits. After breast augmentation, I will see patients yearly for life! This allows for the best care and the detection of any potential problems. There are no charges for any follow up visits. Patients are always encouraged to come to the office at any time for a check up if desired. All patients will also be given my personal cell phone. This provides comfort knowing they can reach the doctor for problems. I recommend texting as a modern and efficient method of communication.

Chapter 3

# The "Do Not Do" List!

It is important to have thorough and comprehensive instructions after cosmetic surgery. My patients get complete postoperative surgical instructions to maximize a safe and easy recovery. They also get my personal cell phone. This is so they can contact me personally if anything happens or questions arise. Despite the complete instructions, patients sometimes have additional questions or thoughts on what to do or not to do.

I believe that extensive postoperative instructions are of paramount importance after your procedure. Complete, thorough, and easy to follow instructions are provided. However, people sometimes do things that are **not** helpful after surgery and can even be harmful. I believe that an important concept after surgery is that patients sometimes make mistakes by doing things that were "not" discussed. Since extensive postoperative instructions are given, these instructions are usually followed and done. It is things that are not discussed that can lead to problems. I describe it as the "Do Not Do" list.

Soaking in a hot tub is a classic mistake after surgery. The soaking can cause infection or injure incisions. Many patients will instinctually know not to do this. But not everyone understands this can be bad. A patient might say to me, "You didn't tell me not to do that!" Because of these questions, I have come up with my "Do Not Do" list. But understand that no list can be 100% complete. No matter how long the list is, there will be something that is not on the list that could be harmful.

A good way to think of postoperative instructions is to follow everything that you are told "to do." Everything else is on the "Do Not Do" list. Remember, all patients are given extensive instructions that are precise on what you should do to maximize recovery! These instructions are complete and are also on my web page. The list that follows is extra things and ideas that can be bad or harmful and should not be done. Instructions, in general, cover what should be done by the patient to recover. This list is what should not be done after surgery. But remember this fact. No list of things can be totally complete. If it is not on the instruction sheet, than consider that it should not be done. Any things that are not mentioned in the instructions should be avoided. This includes instructions from friends who are nurses, medical professionals, or other experts. This includes friends who have had similar operations. If you are in doubt, text me and ask if it is ok to do it. Always remember to ask! By doing this you will be safe. A famous plastic surgeon once said, "Be wise during recovery."

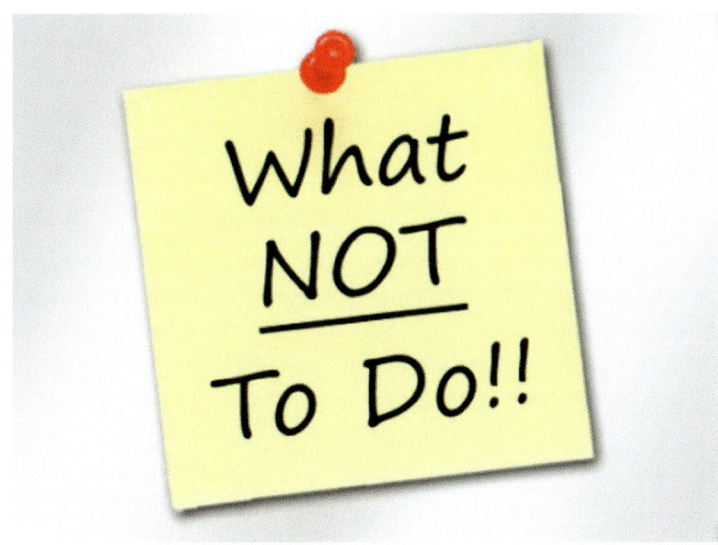

## General Things on the "Do Not Do!" List

No baths or soaking
No hot tubs
No sex
No physical exertion
Don't overdo it
No straining, yelling, pulling, or bearing down
No heating pads or electric blankets to any part of your body, especially surgical areas
Do not apply any lotions, creams, or healing scar treatments until instructed to do so
Don't play with your bandages
Don't stick things underneath your bandages
Don't touch your incisions until told it is safe

### *Specific to Tummy Tucks*

Do not play with or swing around your surgical tubes
Do not touch (within three inches) the entrance site to the drain tube going into your skin
Don't blow into your drains (this goes inside you)
Do not sit or stand in one position for more than 5 minutes
Don't twist your abdomen side to side

### *Specific to Face Lift or Eyelid Surgery*

Don't bend over
Don't put your head below the level of your heart
Don't strain, lift, or pull
Don't get anxious
Don't raise your blood pressure
Don't yell or scream
Don't laugh or talk loudly
Don't rub your eyes
Don't read, watch TV, or keep your eyes open too much - until allowed

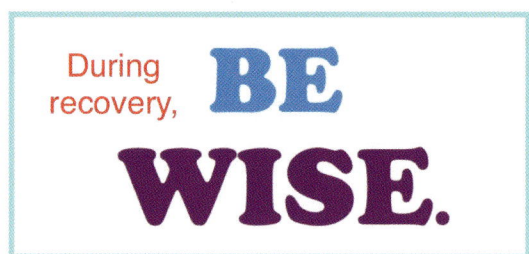

All patients are provided with extensive instructions on what to do after their cosmetic operation. These are also to be found on my web page. Some people will do things after surgery that are not always good for healing and can cause complications. The above list includes many things that are "not to be done" after operations. I call it the "Do Not Do" list. After your cosmetic operation, it is smart to remember - slow and steady wins the race. If you have questions - Ask! All patients have the doctor's personal cell phone. Finally, be smart, be wise, and recover safely.

Chapter 4

# Smoking

Smoking is one of the worst things that a patient can do both before and after surgery. Quitting smoking is extremely important and cannot be over emphasized. If necessary, I will help you with quitting smoking, and there are other resources available to help you do this. This includes most hospitals and primary care physicians will have free programs or services to help an individual quit smoking.

What was just described above about quitting smoking is easy to say, but it is not easy to do. The famous American author Mark Twain said "Quitting smoking is easy to do, I've done it hundreds of times." I personally used to smoke and also used other nicotine products. I tried to quit for 20 years, if not longer, and ultimately was successful. It was probably one of the hardest things I ever did in my life. So I have compassion for the person trying to quit smoking. As I said above, there is probably nothing more important for recovering from cosmetic surgery than quitting smoking.

But it's not just quitting smoking for surgery that is paramount. Quitting smoking is important for your overall health. Smoking leads to hardening of the arteries and atherosclerosis. This can lead to heart attacks, strokes, and peripheral arterial disease. Of course, smoking can also cause mouth, tongue, and oral pharyngeal cancers, in addition to lung cancer. According to the CDC, people who smoke cigarettes are 15 to 30 times more likely to get lung cancer or die from lung cancer than people who do not smoke.

YOUR BODY AFTER YOU STOP SMOKING

**AFTER 20 MINUTES:**
- Blood pressure goes down.
- Heart rate goes down.
- Hands and feet get warmer.

**AFTER 8 HOURS:**
- Blood carbon monoxide levels return to normal.
- Blood oxygen levels go up.

**AFTER 24 HOURS:**
- Heart attack risk is lower.

**AFTER 48 HOURS:**
- Body becomes free of nicotine.
- Nerve endings adjust to missing nicotine.
- Sense of taste and smell start to improve.

**AFTER 72 HOURS:**
- Bronchial tubes start to relax.
- Easier to breathe.

**AFTER 2 -13 WEEKS:**
- Blood circulates better.
- Exercise is easier.

**AFTER 1 YEAR:**
- Heart disease risk is cut in half.

**AFTER 5 YEARS:**
- Cervical cancer risk same as nonsmoker.
- Stroke risk same as nonsmoker.

**AFTER 10 YEARS:**
- Lung cancer risk is cut in half.
- Cancer risk of the mouth, throat, esophagus, and bladder is cut in half.

Sources: American Cancer Society. CDC. Indian Journal of Psychiatry. Smokefree NHS.

When I was in medical school, I remember reading a pathology book that I was studying. This book was probably 2 inches thick and had extremely tiny print. It was extremely indepth medical information. When I was studying, I was reading about a liver disease. The pathology book reviewed who gets the disease, the pathophysiology of disease (which is how it is bad for you) and also the treatment and success rate. I was surprised to see that smoking led to this increased disease of the liver. I thought smoking just caused lung cancer and heart attacks. So I started flipping around to other parts of the book. This included diseases of the skin, the prostate, the bladder, the kidneys, brain, pancreas, the heart and the lungs. To my surprise, every single disease in the book had smoking as a significant causative factor! I was blown away by the realization that smoking didn't just cause a few basic problems or cancer, but it actually *rotted us out to the core* and caused and contributed to almost every medical illness known to mankind. Cigarette smoking can cause cancer almost anywhere in the body. According to the CDC, cigarette smoking can cause cancer of the mouth, throat, esophagus, stomach, colon, rectum, liver, pancreas, larynx, trachea, bronchi, kidney, bladder, cervix, and even blood cancers. I tell this as a medical interest point to help patients understand how bad smoking is. *There is nothing worse a human can do for their body!*

I have helped many patients quit smoking. I am surprised at how quickly they can actually physically look better and feel better. Another interesting thing I learned about quitting smoking was how quickly your risk of diseases drops. Your risks of getting a medical problem can dramatically plummet to near normal levels in relatively short periods of time. It's actually great news for the person quitting smoking. For example, if a patient has smoked for 20 years, they have a much higher chance of lung cancer than the normal population. Remember the risk of lung cancer is not zero for the non-smoker, as even the non-smoker can get lung cancer. But this rate for the non-smoker getting cancer is very low. I think it's extremely important to understand that when you quit smoking, your chance of medical diseases and/or lung cancer actually dramatically plummet! I remember being surprised, and I even thought that it was almost not fair. People that smoke 20 or 30 years could quit smoking, and 1 year later, their risk of lung cancer or heart disease had decreased to extremely and surprisingly low levels. This is actually considered fantastic news. It means that it's never too late to quit smoking. You can really decrease your rate of getting a bad health problem.

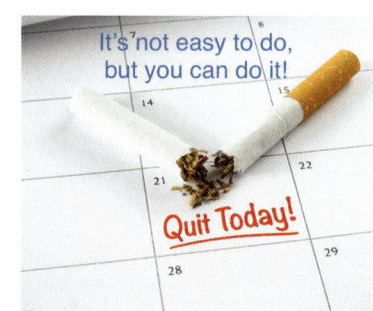

One study in the New England Journal of Medicine found that if you quit smoking by 40, you decrease your chance of dying from smoking related diseases by up to 90%. If you quit by the age of 54, you reduce your chance of dying of smoking related diseases by 66%. If you are older than 54, you can still dramatically decrease your chance of having complications or problems from smoking. *It is never too late to quit!*

I'm going to now talk about some of the pathophysiology of smoking. This means how smoking adversely affects you and recovery from surgery. I used to think it was just because smoking leads to increased coughing. I thought the smoking led to coughing and increased risk of pneumonia. Yes, that can happen after surgery and is one of the reasons why we want to quit smoking. But another reason that might be even more important is how it affects blood supply to the tissues.

Normally, blood travels in our arteries that are essential tubes. These tubes get progressively smaller and smaller. They are called arteries then arterioles then capillaries. The smallest little tubes called capillaries are unimaginably tiny. If you look at the back of your fingernail, you can see the redness of a capillary bed filled with blood. Push on your fingernail and you can see it turn white or blanch. This is because you're pushing the blood out of the capillary system. When the blood is in the capillaries, they are so small that the red blood cells (RBC's) in the blood can barely squeeze through the capillaries. Think of it like a turnstile and only one person from the crowd can go through the turnstile at a single time. The tubes get so small that only one RBC can get through at a time.

As the red blood cells go through this tiny capillary, the oxygen comes off the red blood cells and feeds the surrounding cells. RBCs carry oxygen to the tissues and the cells. This is their purpose. Cells need this oxygen to live. The red blood cells have distensibility or flexibility to allow them to squeeze through the tight capillaries. This is part of the normal process of getting oxygen from the blood and the RBCs to your cells, so they can live and heal.

Smoking hinders the red blood cells from bending and having flexibility. It slows them down, so they can't squeeze through and move oxygen to the capillaries. It is this loss of flexibility of the RBCs by smoking that leads to decreased oxygen getting to the incision and tissues. This is the area of the skin and body that needs the oxygen to heal. This decreased oxygen can lead to actual excessive scarring and necrosis (tissue death) of the skin. It's one of the biggest and scariest risks of cosmetic surgery. I have just described the pathophysiology of why smoking can lead to potential complications and injury of the skin.

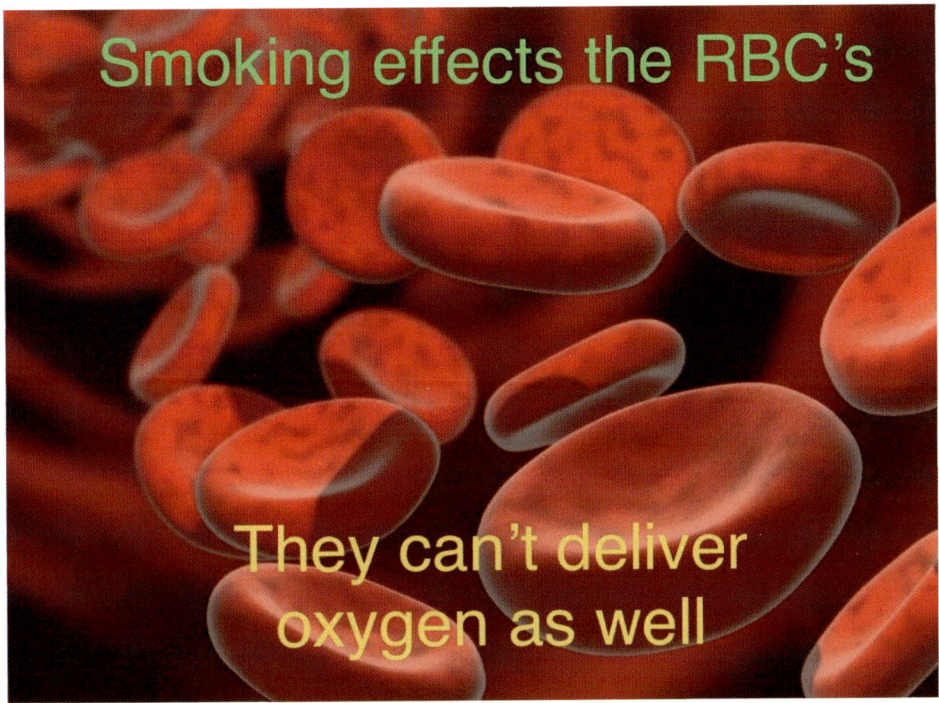

In summary, smoking is extremely bad for all surgery and for the recovery from cosmetic surgery procedures. It is of paramount importance to quit smoking for one month before surgery till one month after surgery. I can help with any of my patients who want to achieve this goal. We only achieve this through hard work and effort. In addition to my help, local hospitals and primary care physicians will also help you with this extremely important task. Keep trying. It's hard. But the effort is necessary to achieve this important task.

Chapter 5

# DVT and Blood Clot Prevention

DVT is the abbreviation for Deep Venous Thrombosis. It is a risk after all operations including cosmetic surgery and plastic surgery. The following chapter will discuss DVT and help a person understand what this is and how we can minimize it happening. This chapter will emphasize DVT from tummy tucks, because this operation is more prone to clots than other cosmetic operations. However, understanding DVT is important for any cosmetic operation. Overall, tummy tuck and cosmetic operations are considered extremely safe! The recommendations in this chapter apply to anyone having any cosmetic operation. We just need to be educated to recover in the safest way possible.

Abdominoplasty is the medical word for cosmetic tummy tuck. This is a wonderful operation that can give a person a flat, tight, and attractive abdominal area. The operation is often part of a mommy makeover and can truly get a woman back into a bikini. This is done by fixing the damages of having babies. It involves improving both the breasts and the stomach at the same time. Results can be amazing!

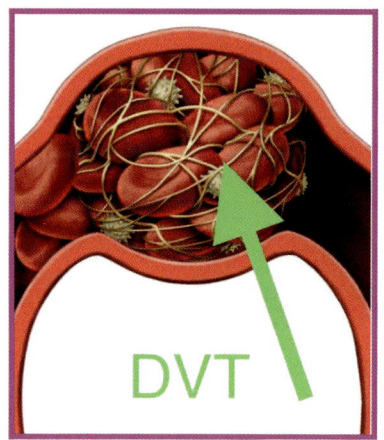

However, like all operations, abdominoplasty surgery does have risks. It is a very safe operation overall. One risk in particular is DVT or deep vein thrombosis. An extremely interesting statistic, in my opinion, is that more than 100,000 people die in America each year from blood clots. This is more than the number of people who die from car accidents and breast cancer combined! This fact underscores the importance of understanding blood clots and the necessity to prevent or minimize the risk of blood clots happening.

After all operations, blood clots or DVT can occur. This tends to occur in the legs right after the induction of anesthesia or the beginning of surgery. The clots are in the deep veins and not the superficial veins that we see on the surface of the legs. If these blood clots occur, there is a risk that they can break off in the veins and travel in the blood to the lungs. This is called a pulmonary embolus or PE. It can be a more serious health issue and hence prevention is important. First, we will discuss risk factors in more detail and then focus on its' prevention- or ways to maximize *not* having this problem.

**Risks Factors:**

All operations have risks of blood clots. People also get blood clots that have not even had surgery. But operations are categorized as being high risk to low risk. High risk procedures in general are not the cosmetic surgery procedures.

These would be operations like cancer operations, pelvic operations, and many orthopedic surgery operations. Plastic surgery procedures are considered low risk. Operations such as facelift, eye tuck, and nose jobs are all considered low risk. Breast augmentation would be another operation that is considered low risk. Tummy tucks, however, are considered more moderate risk. With a moderate risk, we need to be more concerned and emphasize their prevention. But it is always good to focus on blood clot risk with every single operation done.

Risk factors for DVT include but are not limited to:

1- Cancer
2- Birth control pills or hormones
3- Operations
4- High blood viscosity (thick blood)
5- Obesity
6- Obstructed venous return - (vein problems)
7- Lack of movement - (immobility after surgery)
8- Previous DVT
9- Older age

People having cosmetic operations can have some of these risk factors for DVT. However, if you have none of them, it does not mean you will not have a DVT. It just means your risk is much lower. Notice how stopping birth control pills and losing weight are important.

## Prevention:

Many things can be done to decrease our chances of this problem. Active leg exercises, leg elevation, and the use of elastic support stockings can increase vein blood flow and decrease clotting. Early ambulation after surgery and avoidance of prolonged bed rest can promote blood flow and prevent clots. Think of the blood flow in our legs as like a slow moving stream. Anything that improves flow or helps the blood flow helps prevent DVT. Even elevating the foot of the bed 45 degrees can help promote blood drainage. Patient positioning after surgery will be discussed to help us recover safely.

I came up with the acronym "PAIL" to help us remember things to do after surgery to decrease DVT.

## P-A-I-L

P - Positioning:
Keep the "toes above the nose" to help blood flow. A lounge chair is not tilted back enough. The legs are elevated, but they aren't elevated enough. I call it the "tilted back lounge chair." Get the legs up and the chest (where the heart is) down. Use pillows to get those legs way above the heart.

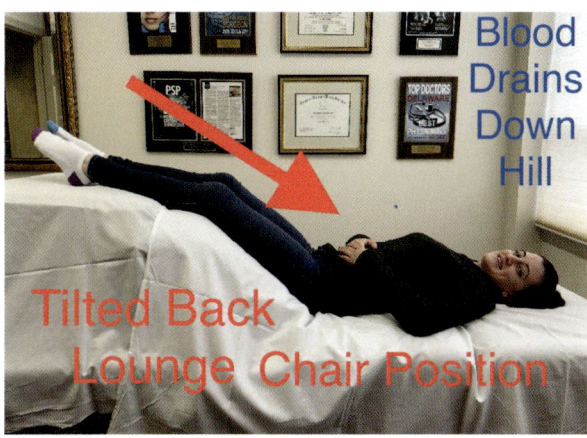

A - Ambulation (early ambulation):
Get out of bed frequently. A minimum of 5-10 times a day for 5-10 minutes each time. More is better. This encourages blood flow. If you are recovering from a tummy tuck, I recommend no twisting of the waist when walking. By avoiding twisting, it encourages the skin to heal to the underlying muscles and decreases fluid accumulation. With other operations, you can twist without risk.

Another way to do early ambulation after surgery is to actually get out of bed and just "march in place." Like a soldier, you can get up and march. Get those knees up high. You don't even have to move. This *marching* promotes the blood movement that minimizes clot risks. For some who are unsteady on their feet after surgery, you can just "march in place!" Early ambulation is critically important after surgery.

I - Invisible Bicycle:

Despite early ambulation, we still have a lot of time in bed. If you are getting out of bed 10 times for 10 minutes, that is still under 2 hours. So we are still in bed about 22 hours after surgery early in the recovery. We can promote blood flow by moving the legs like riding an "invisible bicycle." This can be done in bed with minimal pain after surgery, even an abdominoplasty. You can't do this enough! Do it as much as you can.

The *invisible bicycle* is done one leg at a time. Keep your head rested and back on your pillow, and move one leg at a time. Move it like a bicycle. If the other leg is relaxed and your head is relaxed, the leg will move because of the iliopsoas muscle in the inner back. The abdominal muscles will be relaxed. This will lead you to be able to move the leg easily without hurting the stomach after tummy tuck.

Also, when not doing the bicycle exercise, you can move just the feet. Step on an imaginary gas pedal. Pull the feet back hard. This contracts the calf muscles and promotes blood flow. It must be done **hard** so the muscles really contract. Don't just lightly wiggle them. You also can do this extremely frequently.

L - Leg Compression:

I use sequential leg compression machines for all of my operations to squeeze your legs during surgery and promote blood flow. Leg stocking are recommended, as well, to help with this. Knee high stockings to compress the veins are recommended. These can be purchased at many drug stores and medical supply stores. They are also on-line. They should be of moderate compression, not too loose or too tight.

Wear Compression Stockings

## Summary

Understanding that blood clots are a risk of all cosmetic operations is extremely important. We also want to be aware of different ways we can minimize or prevent blood clots from forming. The acronym *PAIL* is used to help remember important things to do after surgery. Remember "an ounce of prevention is worth a pound of cure." This means try and do all that has been recommended above to try and prevent this problem from happening after cosmetic surgery.

Chapter 6

# Incisions and Scars

## Overview:

For most plastic surgery procedures, it is necessary to have an incision or a "cut." Incisions turn into your scars. These incisions might be very small for liposuction, but they can be long for procedures such as a tummy tuck or a thigh lift. Scars can also come from lacerations, injury, or trauma. Scars can take a year or longer to fade, and this chapter will review the recovery, healing, and treatment of incisions and scars. Sometimes scars can need revisions or operative procedures to make them look better. The patient on the right had a facial scar from a dog bite that was 40 years old. I performed a surgical revision to improve the scar. The bottom 2 pictures show the scar after healing. Surgery helps scars fade and improve, but scars never go completely away.

Always be gentle with your incisions. They are closed with small, delicate, plastic surgery suture material, but this means they could be vulnerable to disruption if someone were to overdo it. As described in detail in chapter 1, remember to *Be the Turtle* during recovery. This means to go slow and take it easy. If you were to overdo it too quickly, you might exceed the tensile strength of the incision. The tensile strength is how strong the incision is and represents how much force is necessary to pull it apart or to disrupt it. Overdoing it can hurt your incision and adversely effect how it looks. It is not common, but I've seen people actually physically pull apart their incisions through having excessive activity too early. This might be exercise too early or other activities such as sex. You will be instructed when it is safe to resume activities as part of the overall recovery from your operation.

## Biology of healing:

Top 6 pics show cheek scar before cosmetic repair

Bottom 2 pics show after repair by Dr. Saunders

As reviewed, tensile strength is a description of the strength of the incision. It correlates closely with the total collagen content of the incision for approximately the first 3 weeks of healing. This collagen is increasing and the tensile strength of your incision is increasing. The collagen level tends to plateau in approximately 3 weeks, but the tensile strength continues to increase as the intermolecular bonding of the collagen improves. This change also involves organization and remodeling of the collagen fibers. The most rapid increase in strength of your incision occurs over the first couple of months. But there is slow increased strength for at least 2 years. The ultimate strength of the incision never quite equals that of the original skin. But for the average person, this is not noticeable.

Of interest is that your scar will continue to heal for the rest of your life. Although for all practical purposes, we only will see healing and fading for about a year or two, the incision actually never stops healing. There is a complicated process of making collagen followed by collagen breakdown. This cycle leads to remodeling and re-organization of the collagen fibers. This is part of the process how the incision has increased tensile strength over time. But the incision never stops doing this, and it is remodeling for the rest of your life.

Vitamin C is part of this process. The collagen is broken down gradually and continuously, and then the body reforms the collagen in a more organized fashion. If we study history and the British sailors of the 1500's and 1600's, it was known that they developed scurvy, which is a vitamin C deficiency. Their incisions or wounds that were 20 years old and totally healed would

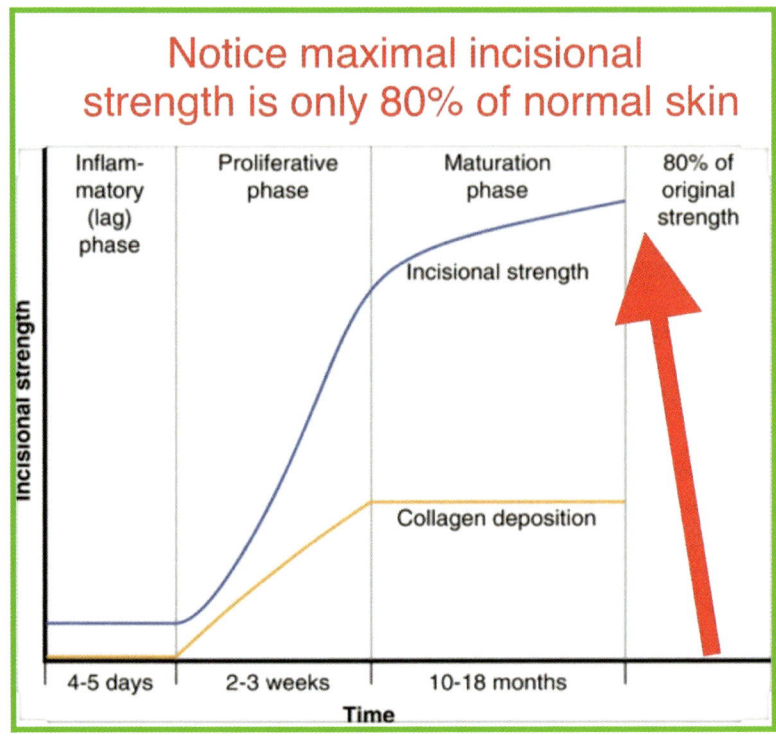

break open as part of the scurvy disease. This is because the body would break down the collagen in the old incision, but needs vitamin C to heal and remodel. Back in this time, scientists did not know what was the cause of scurvy, but they knew that citrus fruits diminished the disease. They didn't know about Vitamin C and how it is necessary to continue healing for your entire life. This is why British sailors would have a supply of citrus, such as limes, on board the ship as they sailed the seven seas. This is the reason a British sailor was called a *limey*.

Many patients ask what vitamins or supplements they can take to help their incision heal. It is not uncommon for doctors to sell or promote certain vitamins and supplements to help the healing process. However, it's been long shown that these do not benefit the average person with a normal diet. If a patient has a normal diet, supplements do not have benefits. This has been shown in hundreds of randomized studies over decades. Supplements of vitamin A, vitamin C, vitamin B complex, and other vitamins do not accelerate or help incisional healing. Interestingly, increasing local oxygen tension with hyperbaric oxygen chambers have been shown to give increased healing of approximately 15 to 20% at 7 days after injury. However, this has been studied extensively and has not been found to be of clinical significance and is not recommended for healthy people with no medical complications. Most importantly, remember that people with a normal diet *do not benefit in any way* from extra vitamins or supplements to heal your incision.

It's normal for incisions to initially have some pleating, swelling, and elevation. The incision is typically surgically closed with three layers of very delicate, fine, and absorbable plastic surgery suture material. It's normal for this absorbable suture to dissolve over a month to two. The incision will often have swelling and show some pleating. This will go away. Do not worry. The swelling is called the "healing ridge." It is normal and to be expected. It goes away.

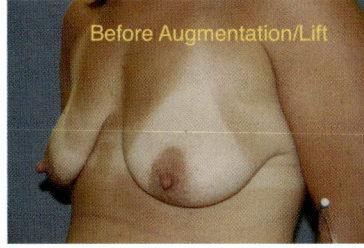 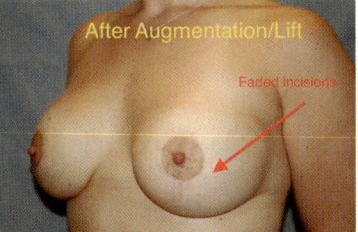 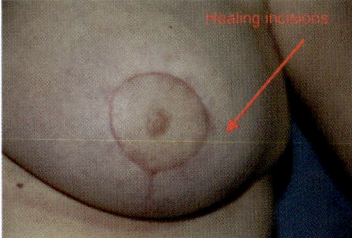

The pictures above show a patient who had surgery by me. The middle picture shows the incisions all faded. The picture on the right shows the incisions when they are still red and fading. The natural healing and fading of the incisions takes approximately a year. Sometimes this can take even 2 years. The vast majority of incisions will fade to a thin line. Incisions do lead to permanent scars. Incisions fade, but they do not completely go away. I, as the plastic surgeon, try to use the most meticulous and delicate techniques to lead to the best fading of the scar.

## Scar Location:

When it comes to real estate, there is an adage "location location location." When it comes to surgical incisions and fading of scars we have the exact same adage. The location is one of the most important factors in the overall healing. Certain locations are privileged and heal extremely well. This includes the face, the eyelids, and around the ears. I describe these areas as being privileged, as they lead to extremely nice scars in the vast majority of circumstances.

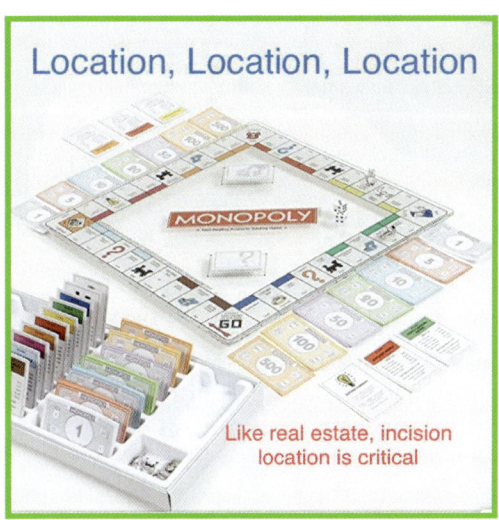

Other locations are not as good as the face. The back is a classic location where scars tend to fade poorly. The extremities often heal less well than desired. With cosmetic operations we choose the incision location, so can have a good understanding of how it will probably fade. This will be reviewed with you during your consultation. It's critically important to understand that some areas heal better than others.

## Scar Care and Treatments

## General Scar Care:

Initially your incision will most likely be covered with Steri-Strips. These are sterile adhesive strips. The Steri-Strips are protective and help the incision heal. They should be removed in 1 week. After removal, I recommend using Neosporin twice a day for 3 days, followed by Bio-Oil twice a day for 3 months. I have had excellent success with

Bio-Oil and recommended it strongly. I consider it a *diamond in the rough.* This is an expression that means it's not expensive, but it works extremely well.

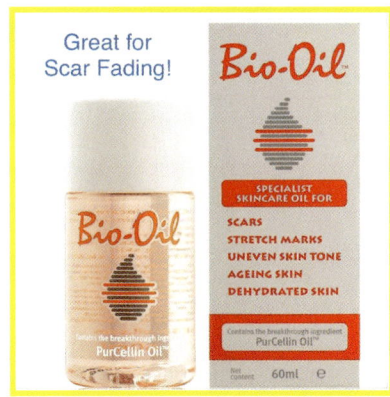

Great for Scar Fading!

Be gentle. Scars can be disrupted. Physical activity that could pull apart your incision should be avoided. Overhead lifting can pull apart arm incisions or breast incisions. Be gentle with leg movements for leg incisions or tummy tucks. Move slowly and carefully. Be wise, because if you don't, you can disrupt things. Initially you should be mainly walking and not lifting above 20 pounds. As you heal, you can gradually increase activity, and this is reviewed with you personally by me depending on your operation.

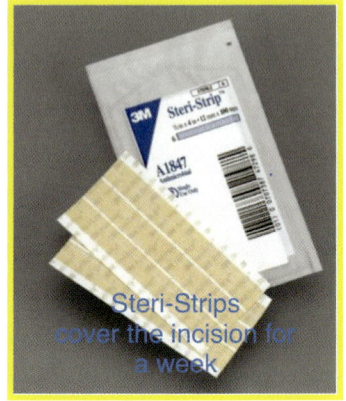

Steri-Strips cover the incision for a week

Don't touch your incision. Hands are not clean.
Hands have touched too many objects and are covered with bacteria. If you touch your incision, you bathe the incision with this bacteria. If you are instructed to remove Steri-Strips or to apply healing creams, first wash your hands well or wear gloves.

Depending on your operation, a binder and/or a garment is worn. The pressure of the garment or binder is extremely important to help healing. The pressure is one of the main factors to help the collagen remodel and the scar to flatten. Burn victims will be given compression garments to promote scar healing. Wear your garment, it will help the scar fade. This is for a year in many cases!

In general, if your scar is healing well, no additional treatments will be necessary other than the ones I just described. But if we are unlucky or have a problem, I will institute additional treatments. I will review some of these now.

**Steroids and Lasers:**

In the unfortunate circumstance of a scar not healing well, different treatments can be instituted. Steroid creams have been shown to be very effective for redness and hardness. This is for prolonged redness, as it's normal to have this for a month or two. This is the period when it gradually fades. If the redness is prolonged and the scar is still hard, it may be hypertrophic. In my opinion, steroids and lasers can help in this circumstance. Steroids can be applied 3 times a day, and I will prescribe one for you. Use it religiously, and don't miss an application.

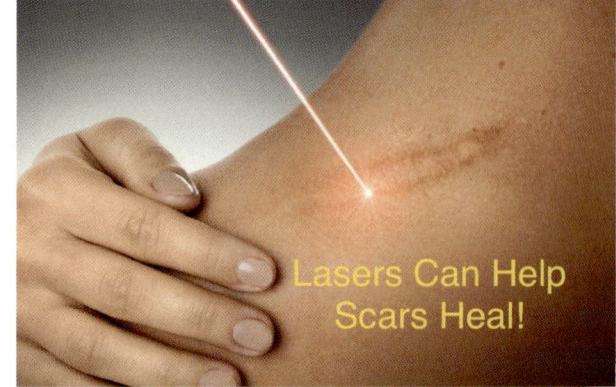

Lasers Can Help Scars Heal!

Laser treatments can be instituted also. IPL lasers can help with the fading of the scar. I have had excellent success with this laser and recommend it for many patients to aid with the healing process. It requires a series of 4 or 5 laser treatments spread out over several months. This is highly effective.

## Silicone Sheets or Creams:

I used to recommend silicone strips and silicone creams. I found these to be overpriced, labor intensive, and also not that effective. However, if somebody has had success with them in the past, then I recommend to use them again. This is because every individual is unique, and prior success would change my recommendation to use what was successful before.

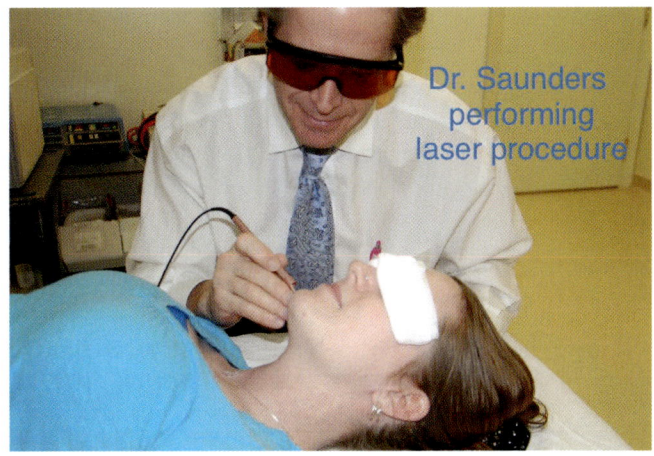

Dr. Saunders performing laser procedure

## Massage:

Scar massage can be done to help your scar heal and fade. Scar massage is the process of manually rubbing and pushing on your scar. It is typically done for approximately 10 to 20 minutes 10 times a day. It is a labor intensive treatment. I often recommend doing it more frequently at night, when you're watching TV and relaxing. Don't press on the scar too hard. It should be more of a moderate force. Excessive force could cause bruising and injury. Pressing too lightly will do nothing. A moderate force gives the best result, and this will be shown to you personally by me during your follow up visit to the office.

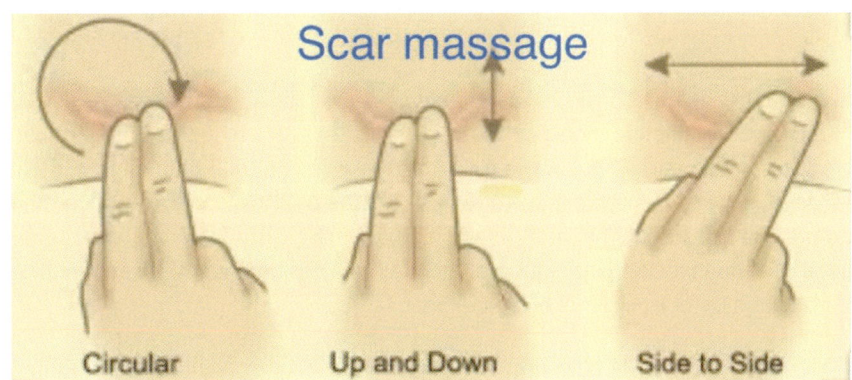

Scar massage

Circular | Up and Down | Side to Side

Chapter 7

# The Pain Buster or Pain Pump

## Summary

The Pain Buster is a postoperative medicine delivery machine that provides continuous pain medicine directly to the surgical site. It gives amazing and unparalleled pain control. This small machine has, in my opinion, revolutionized the recovery and post-operative pain management after many cosmetic operations. In particular, breast augmentation recovery and tummy tuck recovery are the main operations where it is used. The recovery has become so much better and with less pain, that many patients often can not believe how easy it is to heal. This chapter will review how the Pain Buster or pain pump works and why it makes such a big difference when recovering from plastic surgery.

## What is the Pain-Buster, and What Does it Look Like?

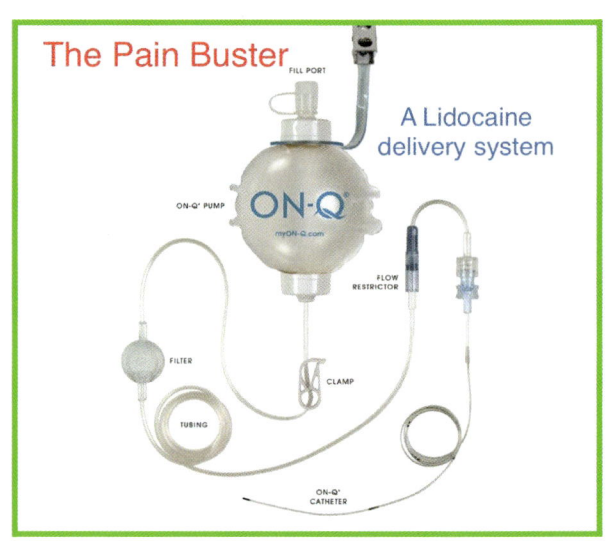

The Pain Buster is a medical device to give a patient a continuous stream of extremely safe numbing medicine. The goal of the device is to provide unparalleled control of pain after surgery. The Pain Buster delivers a safe local anesthetic (Lidocaine) directly to the area where it is needed. This means directly to the stomach muscles for an abdominoplasty or directly beneath the muscle for breast enlargement. The delivery of the medicine is for 72 hours or 3 days. Most of the pain after the operations is for this time period. Hence the device gets the patient through and past the worst part of the recovery period. It really gets you over the hump until you are feeling much better. It is not a PCA or patient controlled anesthesia machine. These devices deliver narcotics like morphine into the vein. This can be dangerous because of overdose and side effects. This pump delivers lidocaine. It's so safe you can actually drink the medicine.

This pain delivery system looks like a compact and neat medicine ball. It is pictured above. The patient wears a fanny pack around their waist, that contains the medicine reservoir. This reservoir is round or cylindrical in shape. The medicine is placed into this holding area. Out of the reservoir comes a tiny tube that splits into two tubes. These are extremely small and leave no scar. The tubes have a series of holes at the end that allow the medicine to come out into the desired location. There is a regulator at the beginning of the tube that controls how much medicine comes out at any time. There is also a clip that clamps the tube off, that allows it to be shut off if needed. The device is not adjustable. You can not turn it up or down. It is fully automatic.

## How Does the "Pain Buster" Work, and What is the Medicine?

The Pain Buster works by a pressure gradient. The ball or reservoir is filled and has a higher pressure than the area inside the breast or abdomen. The regulator allows for the correct amount of medicine to be infused slowly and safely. The pressure change leads to the medicine slowly trickling into the desired location for pain control. A regulator controls how much medicine is delivered. This usually means that about 2-4 cc of lidocaine is delivered per hour. The reservoir ball is connected to the patient by two tubes. These tubes are extremely tiny. As I have described, they leave no scar.

The tubes are placed at the time of the cosmetic operation under sterile conditions. The tubes deliver the medicine to the location needed. They have lots of little holes at the end, so the medicine trickles out over a wider area. I describe it like a tiny garden "soaker hose." The tubes allow for the medicine to slowly come out and soak or bathe the muscles, giving fantastic pain control.

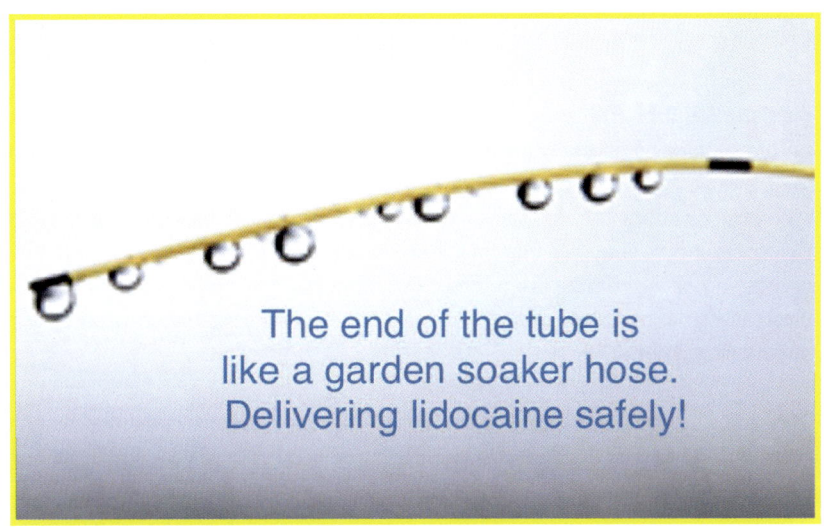

The end of the tube is like a garden soaker hose. Delivering lidocaine safely!

The Pain Buster is filled with a medicine that most people have heard about because of its use in dentistry. The active ingredient is lidocaine, also known as Xylocaine. It was first made by a Swedish chemist named Nils Lofgren. His partner first used it on himself in 1949, and he documented its' incredible safety. Lidocaine has a proven track record of well over 70 years. The medicine is not a narcotic, which underscores its' safety.

## What are the Advantages to Using it, and Which Operations Work Best with it?

Medical studies with the Pain Buster have shown a more comfortable recovery, quicker return to normal activities, greater mobility, clearer thinking, and faster return to normal bowel habits after surgery. The main advantage is less pain and a continuous infusion of a non-narcotic medication. Narcotics can cause nausea, vomiting, constipation, malaise, and confusion. They also have tolerance, which means that it works less well with time. The Pain Buster and the extreme safety of lidocaine have led to an incredible reduction in the postoperative pain after surgery. It has in my opinion revolutionized the recovery from many operations. The days of hospitals and IV morphine are long gone! The pain reduction is often fantastic, as I have stated. But, it is important to understand that it doesn't work perfectly for everyone. Some patients will have more pain than desired, and it is common to still supplement the pain management with oral pills such as Percocet and/or Vicodin. It is also ok to add Tylenol or Motrin if needed.

The best operations to use this pump for are breast augmentation and tummy tuck. It is also used when both operations are done together. This is called a *mommy makeover*. The lidocaine infusion works wonderfully for breast implants by bathing the muscle area providing fantastic relief. For the abdominoplasty, the lidocaine trickles into the muscle repair and leads to a quicker and easier recovery. I can not overemphasize how much this device has revolutionized the recovery from these operations.

Chapter 8

# Nutrition and Diet for Cosmetic Surgery

## Summary

Many patients have questions before and after cosmetic surgery that focus on nutrition and diet. How do I best lose weight? What is the best diet? What exercise program is recommended? Cosmetic surgery patients often ask for information on nutrition after their procedure.

Nutrition has always been one of my extra interests. I have studied nutrition for over 30 years and have been a published author on human metabolism and nutrition. My recommendations are based on doctor studies *by doctors* and *for doctors*. It is essential information that is accurate and most importantly honest.

Many informational sources on nutrition in fitness magazines, print, or the Internet are skewed to sell something or to be promotional. They are trying to make it unique and interesting. Often there are hidden financial reasons to sell something or to promote something. For example, the nut industry is over 50 billion dollar business a year. They get people and "experts" to promote nuts to make money, and often what they are saying is inaccurate or slanted.

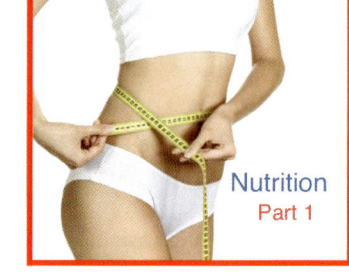

Nutrition
Part 1

This chapter will give you the real *skinny*. No pun intended. It will review critical nutrition and diet information that will help you with your cosmetic surgery but also for a life-time of health.

This chapter is divided into two parts. Part One focuses on general concepts for nutrition and diet. Part Two focuses on more specific nutrition and dietary guidelines and issues.

## Part One : General Concepts

### Exercise Regularly and Don't Eat Crap:

Many people are looking for the easy way out. The diet that "tricks" the body and leads to weight loss without hard work. Diets are hard work for most people. There are no tricks. You can not eat *crap* food and be sedentary and have significant weight loss. Many scientific studies have shown that fad diets don't last, and I do not recommend them.

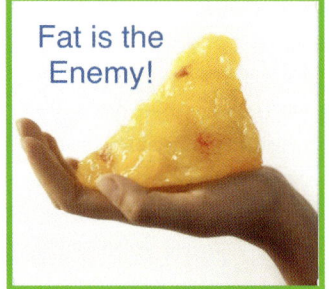

Fat is the Enemy!

Exercise regularly and don't eat crap! This is the diet after cosmetic surgery that will work for most people. This is the diet plan and nutrition that has been shown to work. It's not easy. It's hard. But it is often extremely successful.

### Fat is the Enemy:

The goal of many cosmetic surgery operations is to be made smaller and thinner. Liposuction, tummy tuck, and many operations target fat and fat cells. The operations try to achieve significant reductions in fat cells and volume. However, the best results are when the patient understands there are limitations to what surgery can do. Diet, exercise, and nutrition can take us further and make the results even better. Diet and exercise begin where surgery stops. It is extremely important to understand that diet and exercise are part of the best cosmetic surgery results. After surgery I help my patients with coordinated plans to lose weight and get healthier. This is called a cosmetic surgery nutrition plan.

## Outside Fat is the Tip of the Iceberg:

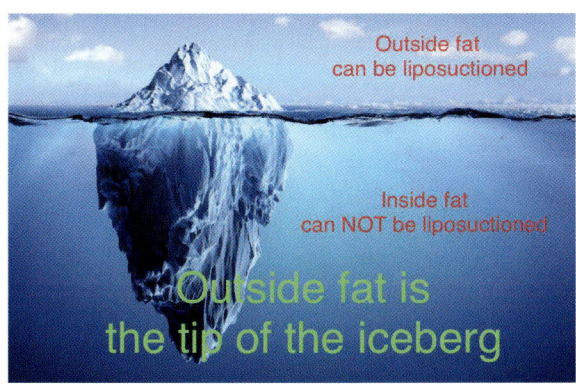

People interested in nutrition after cosmetic surgery often ask how much weight they are going to lose after the procedure. Questions often focus on how many pounds will be removed after liposuction of the stomach, or how much weight will be lost after a tummy tuck. Many people will be surprised by the answer. It's often much less than you would believe. They might love their result and the way they look after their cosmetic operation, but they can be surprised about the actual weight loss. Most of our weight is inside us and not outside. Liposuction patients might lose only a pound or two. Tummy tuck patients will say that their stomach weighs 10 pounds. Most of the time it is only 3-5 pounds.

The knowledge that most of our weight is inside us is important. Outside fat is just the tip of the iceberg. To repeat, most of our fat is inside us and accounts for the majority of our fat. Significant weight loss after surgery usually leads to much more dramatic results. After surgery is often the best time to get the weight off and *go for it!*

## Why the Focus on Fat?

There are two main reasons for this. Fat has 9 calories per gm of food. Protein and carbohydrates (carbs) have about 4-5 calories per gm. This means you have to burn off double the amount of calories for fat as compared to protein and carbs. This is a huge difference. If you eat 100 gm of pure carbs, you will have to burn off about 400 calories to stay even. Eat 100 gm of fat and you have to burn off 900 calories! This is a huge difference.

Fats are compacted energy sources biologically and chemically. They are our body's storage source for when we have no food. Eating fat means eating double the amount of calories, and you will have to burn off double the amount to stay even. This is why fats are so important to monitor in any diet after cosmetic surgery.

Another reason is that diets focused on fat reduction have been shown to have high and long term success. Like Weight Watchers and LA Diet programs, counting of calories and fat can really *work* for the long run. Medical study after medical study have shown that *fad* diets often have high rebound weight gain after short periods of time.

## Weight Loss and Surgery:

Patients might have heard that all weight loss before a tummy tuck should be done before the operation. This is not the whole story. Weight loss before the operation is recommended, but weight loss afterwards is also highly successful too. Weight loss before is thought to be the best, because all the extra skin will be present at the operation. However, the problem with this approach is that many people can't lose weight before and that is why they want cosmetic surgery to begin with.

For people who are having problems losing the weight before their operation, losing it afterwards works fantastic. Many people get motivated after surgery. They have spent money, recovered, and seen the benefit of the operation. They don't want to ruin it. Many people feel more comfortable in their workout clothes after surgery and now succeed in weight loss. Any weight loss after surgery only makes things better. If you lose 5-20 pounds after your operation, you are just going to look even better and more sculpted. It usually doesn't create excess skin, it makes you thinner and *enhances* the results.

Weight loss after liposuction is the same situation. Proper nutrition after liposuction can help a person lose weight. This, in most situations, leads to *improved* results. It gets rid of extra fat that wasn't removed. It leads to enhanced results and increased satisfaction with the operation. The answer usually is lose weight. Proper diet and nutrition are the ways we enhance results after cosmetic surgery.

## Part Two : Nutrition and Dietary Guidelines

As discussed above, there are no tricks or fad diets that work well. Diet after cosmetic surgery or diets in general are hard work and require effort. I recommend a strong attitude and continued effort to achieve the best weight loss and diet. Exercise regularly and don't eat crap. This is a good overall motivating phrase. As part of a comprehensive cosmetic surgery nutrition plan, I will give now sound tips and things to avoid.

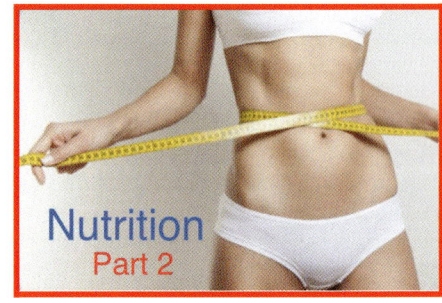

Overall, keep in mind wise and intelligent advice for proper nutrition and diet.

1 - Eat and drink smart:
Watch out for poor foods high in calories. Be careful of too much alcohol, soda, and other high calorie drinks.

2 - Exercise regularly:
Regular exercise burns calories and promotes health. It is good for the heart, blood pressure, and just about everything else. Mental health is dramatically helped by regular exercise.

3 - Get educated on food:
This information source is done to help you with this process. It is actually easy. Soon you will know what to look out for and what is healthy food.

4c- Try and try again:
Like quitting smoking, keep up the effort to lose weight. Don't give up. With perseverance most people will succeed.

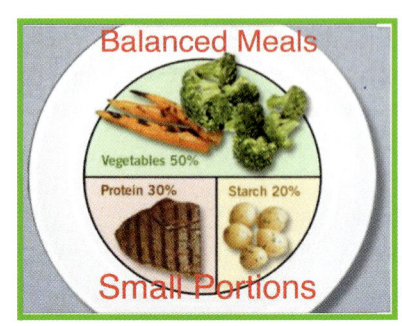

5 - Doctors and programs:
There are doctors who do nothing but help you with diet and weight loss. Programs are readily available which will increase your chance of success.

Watch these misleading things that can trick you. A good diet plan should focus on learning information that *isn't* correct. A lot of nutritional advice is not good nutritional information. Here are 7 important ones.

1 - Antioxidants:
This has been a big advertising campaign from many food sellers. From green tea to certain nuts, diets high in antioxidants are claimed to be healthy and promote longer life span. Multiple major medical studies published in medical journals and the Journal of Epidemiology have shown this to be *false*. The studies show that antioxidants gave zero benefit when compared to people with normal diets. If you eat normally and are not malnourished, foods with added antioxidants have no added value for us.

2 - Zero grams trans fat:
Advertisements for food and labels can be misleading. The idea is that lower levels of "bad" fat are better. Trans fat or saturated fats are less healthy than unsaturated ones. However, this doesn't mean the fat content isn't high. Some foods are horribly high in fat but low or zero in trans fat. These foods are not healthy, and you should not be tricked by it. *Look at total fat content.* This is the key number.
Two examples follow:

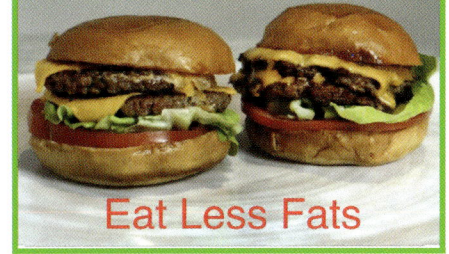

i - Cheetos - zero trans fat. However total fat is 24gm or 48% of your daily recommended fat.
ii - Lays Potato Chips - zero trans fat. However total fat is 27gm or 54% of your daily recommended fat.

3 - Beware of low or fat free food advertisements:
There are other foods with similar claims to what was just described above. Fat is important, but calories can make you fat too. For example, soda, beer, alcohols, and pasta can add significant calories. They have little to no fat but are packed with calories. Remember, cows get fat on grass. Grass has no fat. They just eat way too much.

4 - Watch snacks:
Potato chips and tortilla chips have a high fat content. Some have 1 gm per chip. Think how many chips can be eaten as an appetizer even before you start your meal. If you eat 10 chips, this is 10 gms of fat = 20% of your daily recommended fat. And it's just a snack.

5 - Watch most fast foods and fried foods:
The foods at fast food restaurants often are extremely high in fat and calories. A hamburger and french fries can be over 1000 calories and over 100% of fat for the day. It's only one meal!

6 - Low carb diets often don't work:
Stick to diets that count total calories and fat. Carbs should make up about 40-60% of your diet. Low carb diets are not recommended by me, and they can be nutritionally unwise with deficiencies. Also, they tend to be part of fad diets that don't work well or maintain benefits of weight loss. Carbs should be a huge part of our daily diet. But the carbs should be vegetables and fruits, and they should not be candy, white bread, and beer. Carbs are always the biggest source of our daily diet in doctor recommended sources and diets.

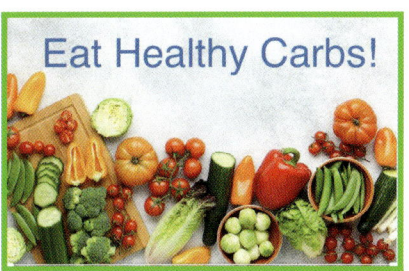

7 - Try to cut refined sugars or empty carbs:
Coke, sodas, candies, and cakes are almost pure sugar. They are empty calories with little nutrients.

**Remember these 5 facts to help with general health, nutrition, and diet after cosmetic surgery:**

1 - Watch soda!
High in calories and without any nutrition.
2 - Cut fast foods and eating out!
High in calories and fat. Many hidden calories.
3 - No super sizes and watch out for large portions!
Guaranteed to get way too much fat and calories.
A large French fries at Mcdonald's is 500 calories and 25 gms of fat!
4 - Minimize snacks!
Potato chips, cookies, dips, and many snacks are fat promoting.
It also is a bad habit or "eating behavior."
5 - Get moving.
Exercise! Burn calories. Be healthy.

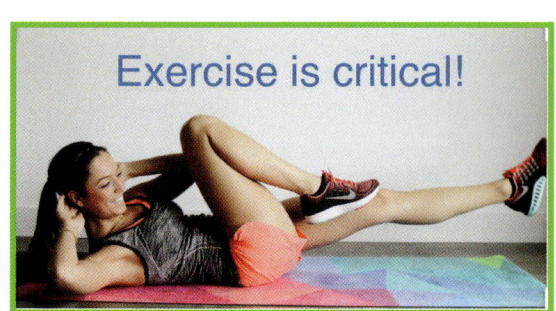

**Eating behaviors:**
Good habits are important to learn. Bad habits are tough to break!

1 - Don't eat and watch tv. Eat at the table only.
2 - Eat slowly.
3 - Don't buy *bad* food items. i.e. (potato chips, candies, or fatty foods)
4 - Buy good snacks and small sizes.
5 - Plan meals.
6 - Watch urges.
7 - *Say no!* You don't need the second margarita or that dessert.

**Keep a food and exercise journal:**
This is extremely helpful to figure out if your diet and exercise program is working. Record everything. This allows adjustments to get better weight loss and stability.

1 - Record diet and exercise.
2 - Develops control - *Try to not eat or refraining.*
3 - Prevents forgetting what has been eaten.
4 - Motivates.

To begin a diet after cosmetic surgery or to begin any nutritional diet plan, we focus on total calories and total fat goals. I like starting with 1500 calories and 50 gms of fat for women. For men, I recommend 2000 calories and 50 gms of fat. 50 gms of fat is a great goal, because the amount eaten in a meal or snack can be doubled to give an easy percentage of daily fat intake. For example, if you eat large french fries at McDonald's, you eat 25 gms of fat. Double this and you find that you have just eaten 50% of your total daily fat!
The 1500 calories is a starting point. It can be adjusted up or down depending on your results. Your journal should cover detailed exercise as well. If you exercise more, your allowed calories will go up.

**Remember:** Eat like a queen for breakfast, a princess for lunch, and a commoner for dinner. Studies have shown that late night meals and big dinners are associated with significant weight gain. Eating earlier in the day allows for your body to more naturally burn off the calories and leads to weight loss.

Chapter 9

# Recovery in an Outpatient Surgery Center

I perform almost all of my operations in a deluxe outpatient surgical facility. The facility is called the Brandywine Cosmetic Surgery Center. It is an outpatient facility that specializes in exclusively cosmetic surgery. Other names for this type of facility include same day surgical facility and outpatient surgical facility. They are commonly called a surgery center or surgicenter abbreviated.

The Brandywine Surgery Center is a state licensed, deluxe, cosmetic surgery center. I perform almost all of my cosmetic procedures in this facility. The center was designed and built using all state guidelines and safety features. It has every safety feature of a hospital without exception. It is also much cleaner than a hospital ever could be. Many patients have commented that it is like a small deluxe hospital. One of the most important features of the center, as I have said, is its' cleanliness. Since it is personally run and managed by me, the facility is extremely clean and immaculate. On operative days, it is often cleaned up to 7 separate times. This is, in my opinion, a major advantage over a hospital. Hospitals are communal in their very nature. Hospitals have higher infection rates. Major bacteria such as MRSA, VRE, and super resistant bacteria are probably unlikely in my clean surgicenter. These are more frequent problems in hospitals and are called *nosocomial* infections. Most people understand that surgery centers are vastly cleaner. I, however, cannot promise or guarantee that there won't be an infection. This would be unlikely, however. We do our best to have the best operation in the cleanest, safest, and healthiest environment.

The surgery center also allows me to control all other factors going into your operation. My nurses and staff are hand picked and specially trained. They are educated on the intricacies and the specialized details of cosmetic surgery. The surgical assistance and anesthesia team are all experts in helping cosmetic surgery. Controlling all of these factors allows me to focus on the surgery at hand to maximize its chance of success.

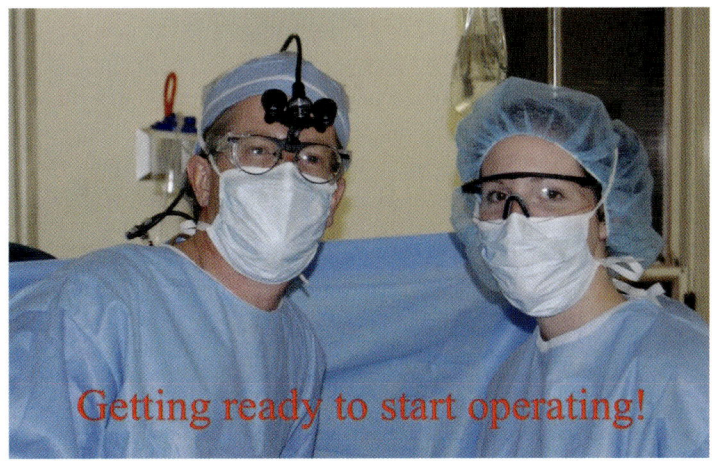
Getting ready to start operating!

Chapter 10

# Breast Augmentation

## Summary

Breast augmentation or breast enlargement is one of the most commonly performed operations in America. Approximately 350,000 women have breast enlargement each year. It is a wonderful operation with high satisfaction and success rates. It can often give patients the breasts they have only dreamed about. I have always been amazed at the incredible depth of satisfaction women get with enhanced and fuller breasts. The operation can give patients, in addition to prettier breasts, a confidence and internal satisfaction that is extremely profound and long lasting.

This operation is performed not only on young women in their 20's, 30's and 40's but also by women who have become deflated from children or aging. Women in their 50's, 60's, and 70's will do breast augmentation and exclaim, "Why didn't I do this operation years ago?" The recovery can be under a week for many women with the use of the powerful Pain Buster to help with discomfort.

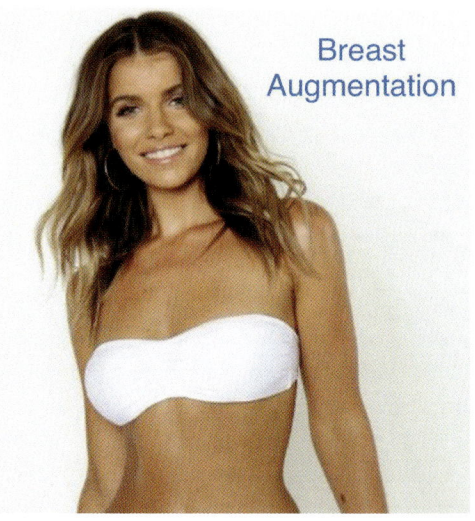

Breast Augmentation

Consultations in my office are extremely thorough and complete. *Homework* is how I term the effort and tasks that we do to help pick the right size implant. This usually means not too big and not too small.

I specialize in this operation. I am a member of the LEAD society. This stands for leadership, education, and development in breast augmentation surgery. I have presented my research at meetings in Montreal and Los Angeles. This chapter will review the recovery from breast augmentation.

## Bandages:

After surgery the patient is bandaged with Steri-Strips on the incisions, a gauze covering, and an ace wrap bandage. It is personally placed by me at the time of surgery. It might feel tight, which is normal. Many doctors use surgical bras which I have found to be "one size fits no one." I feel my ace wrap is perfect. Please do not disrupt or take off the bandage, as this could risk exposing the incision and increase possible infection.

It is common to feel the bandages are a bit tight, because the implants are placed beneath the muscle. This leads to a tight feeling. This includes a feeling of pressure and pain. If for some reason the bandage does become disrupted, please re-wrap the breasts with the ace wrap. Try not to touch the incision or where the Pain Buster comes out of the skin. Hands must be washed or you should wear gloves.

The bandage is typically changed and rewrapped the day after surgery, during your office visit. This is when you get to see your breasts for the first time. The bandage is worn for 3 days, until your first shower. After your shower, you switch to a sports bra which is reviewed below.

**Bleeding:**

It is common to have spotting of blood on the side of the bandage. This is normal. Please do not be alarmed. The pain pump leaks some of the medication out as well. This leakage also contributes to spotting on the sides of the bandage. One side always has more drainage and bleeding than the other. As described above, the bandages are changed the morning after surgery.

**Showering:**

At 72 hours or 3 days, you can take your first shower. You can remove the ace wrap and gauze, but you should leave the Steri-Strips in place. They should be removed approximately 1 week after surgery. Some doctors will say to leave them on for 1 month, but I believe this is old-fashioned. They should be removed at 1 week. After removal of the Steri-Strips, please use Neosporin twice a day for 3 days, followed by Bio Oil twice a day. Showers are allowed daily after the 72 hour period. Bathing and hot tubs are to be strictly avoided.

**The Pain Pump or Pain Buster:**

The Pain Pump or Pain Buster delivers a continuous stream of lidocaine for 3 days or 72 hours. I think this machine has revolutionized the recovery from this operation! It is fantastic to help diminish pain. Lidocaine is so safe you can actually drink it. But remember, the Pain Buster works great, but this does not mean you will have *no pain*. It is automatic and cannot be adjusted to increase the rate. Try not to disrupt or pull out the tubes. If this accidentally happens, please use the white clip inside the fanny pack to stop the flow of medication. Please also read Chapter 7 which describes and shows the Pain Buster in great detail.

**Medications:**

Chapter 2 describes in detail medications to be used after elective cosmetic surgery procedures. The antibiotics are mandatory to take. Intravenous antibiotics are given prior to surgery for prophylaxis and to minimize risks of infection. The oral antibiotics should be started when you get home. If your stomach is upset, they can be started in the morning.

Additional medications include prescriptions for pain, nausea or vomiting, and anxiety. The anxiety medicine also is an antispasmodic medicine. It can be taken in addition to the pain pills for those who need extra pain relief. Motrin and Tylenol also can be added for pain, if needed. Finally, ice application can help. But don't ice directly on the bare skin; cover the ice with a towel or washcloth.

The anxiety medicine is Valium. This medicine also happens to be good for spasms as an antispasmodic. If you are having extra pain, the Valium will work well mixed with the pain pills to give additional pain relief. I would stagger them versus taking them all at the same time. This means taking the pain medication and approximately two hours later taking the Valium, and then another two hours later you take more pain pills. This could also be described as alternating the medication.

In general, pain medications are better tolerated if taken with food. This will mean less nausea and vomiting for those who suffer from this side effect of the pain pills. It is also safe to take Motrin as another medication to help relieve pain. As described the medicines should be staggered and taken at separate times.

**One Side is Different!**

With breast surgery, one breast will always recover, feel, and even look different than the other. It is exceedingly common to feel that one breast is more bruised, swollen, and painful than the other. Also, it is normal to feel one breast is higher, harder, and different than the opposite side. If you do one hundred breast augmentations, one hundred people will feel these differences and describe differences. The plastic surgeon describes this as the breasts are *sisters not twins.*

After and during recovery, it is exceedingly common to notice differences. It can cause people a lot of anxiety. But please be reassured. Breasts settle and drop slightly differently, as muscles on one side are often stronger than the other. Recovery in general differs from side to side. Womens' breasts are usually slightly different before surgery, and this is common afterwards too. Even the final result is typical to have slightly different breasts. Remember, it's described as *sisters not twins.*

**Settling:**

Settling is the process of the tissues and muscles surrounding the implants gradually stretching out after surgery. This process is also called *dropping.* When they are first placed, the muscle and tissue are tight, and the implants tend to be high. Sometimes this is called *high and tight.* The settling process happens gradually over 3 to 6 months. Most people however tend to look significantly settled or improved over just the first 2 to 4 weeks. The settling process is described in more detail in Chapter 12.

**Massage:**

Massage or implant displacement are techniques used to help the breasts soften and to settle. There are two main massage techniques. This includes a pushing from the side and also a pinching technique from the top of the breast. The massage techniques are described in detail in Chapter 11.

A video demonstrating massage is on my webpage at ChrisSaundersMD.com. You should begin these massages after I have reviewed them with you. It is important to understand that many patients will settle normally and will **not** need to do massage. If your implants are staying high, then the massage techniques become more important. The next paragraph reviews shoulder and posture exercises that are important and can assist settling.

**Shoulder Exercises and Posture:**

Because breast implants cause pain, it is common for people to assume a forward appearing or slouched posture. It's a normal splinting mechanism that the body does when it suffers pain in the chest area. This posture, however, can contribute to a higher location of the implants and can hinder the settling process.

By assuming a shoulder down and shoulder back position, we can help with the settling and dropping of the implants. This exercise and posture will be described and shown to you in detail after surgery by me. By placing the shoulders down and back, it stretches the pectoralis muscle. This leads to a gradual stretching of the surrounding tissue and improvement of the appearance and location of the implants. It is done 10 times a day, and the position is held for 2 minutes.

**Return to Work:**

Most people can return to work and light activity after 3 to 5 days. One week off of work, however, is nice for many people and is typical. If you have a job that is manual and requires strenuous activity, then please follow the instructions below under **exercise and activity.**

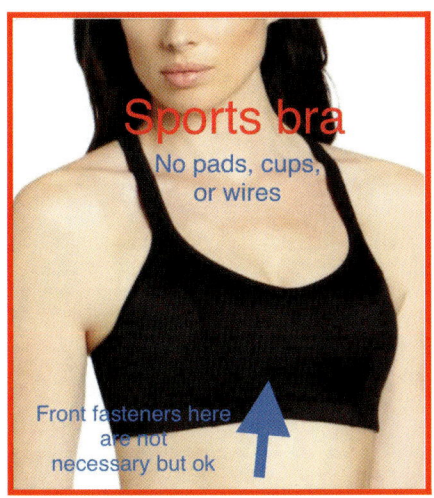

**Bras:**

Sports bras should be worn after your first shower at 72 hours. The sports bra should be an old fashioned sports bra, which means no cups, wires, or padding. It can have front fasteners, but this is not necessary. It should be snug and not too tight or

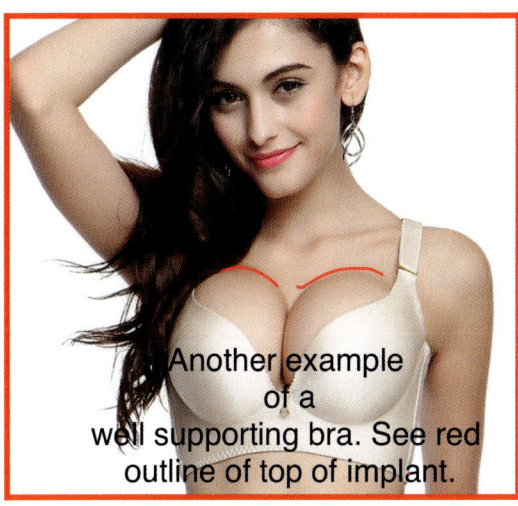

loose. Most sports bras are typically worn for approximately 1 month. After this time, when approved by me, you can switch to any bra desired, including ones with wires.

**Incisions:**

The incision is sewn up with small, inside, pretty plastic surgery stitches. These are all absorbable, so no stitches need to be removed. Steri-Strips are used to cover the incision. These are sterile. They should be removed at 1 week. After the Steri-Strips are removed, Neosporin is used twice a day for 3 days followed by Bio Oil twice a day. I've had great success with this product. I think it's a diamond in the rough, which means that it is inexpensive but highly effective. Patients who want to use silicone strips or silicone creams are allowed to do so. I've used these products for over 20 years. I found them to be expensive and not as effective as Bio Oil. However, if someone has had success with them in the past, then it is a good idea to stick with what has worked for you. Otherwise, please use the Bio Oil to help the incisions fade.

**Exercise and Activity:**

Initially, exercise and activity should be very light. This usually means walking around the home for the first week. You can drive when you feel you can drive safely and defensively. You need to be responsible for your own actions and driving. From 1 week to approximately 1 month, we have what I call a *phased-in* activity period. This means that we're gradually increasing our activity. At 1 month almost anything can be done. Usually after approximately 1 or 2 weeks, depending on your healing, we can resume easy activities such as stationary bicycles, ellipticals, and walking on the treadmill. These activities allow a person, who wants to get some exercise, to get their heart rate up and feel better. It is ok, because it won't affect the breasts healing. Strenuous activities like CrossFit, running, and weightlifting are held off until approved by me, approximately 1 month after surgery.

Chapter 11

# Breast Augmentation Massage

## Summary

What is breast augmentation massage? What is this, and what does it have to do with cosmetic breast implants? Breast augmentation massage is also called implant displacement. It is a series of maneuvers or techniques used to move the implants around inside the body. The purpose is to help stretch out the tissues and to help soften everything after surgery. It also helps to minimize scarring that can sometimes happen in the future. This will be discussed in more detail below. I have a video on my web page which helps review massage and how it is done. The web page is ChrisSaundersMd.Com.

## Why Do We Do These Exercises?

The first purpose of breast massage is to help the breasts and tissues stretch. The tissue and muscle on top of the breast implants will be swollen and *tight* after surgery. This tissue will gradually soften and stretch over time. The swelling will also gradually resolve as part of breast augmentation recovery. Massage will help this stretching process through physical movement and range of motion exercises. Massage will also help with swelling by increasing lymphatic drainage.

The second purpose of breast augmentation massage after surgery is to help minimize scarring in the future. This is called capsular contracture or "hardening of the implants." The idea is that massage after surgery will minimize this scar from forming. It is like stretching to minimize stiff joints. It is analogous to physical therapy after orthopedic or knee surgery. You typically are sent to a physical therapist to help with range of motion and to minimize the risk of scar tissue formation or a stiff knee. After breast surgery, there is no physical therapist. Just you and me. The breast massage helps the healing and helps prevent internal scar tissue that can form.

It has been shown in medical studies of breast augmentation that implants placed beneath the muscle have lower levels of scar tissue formation. It is thought that the muscle may create *internal* massaging. As the muscle contracts, it moves the implant around and leads to decreased scar tissue formation! Massage done by the patient is also believed to decrease this scar tissue from occurring.

## How are They Done?

Breast implant massage exercises are recommended by me after cosmetic breast surgery. During recovery, you will be shown how this is done. It is a two step process. The first is "pushing" from the sides and the second is "pinching" from the top. Both parts are held for several minutes or so and then repeated multiple times a day. Please see my video that shows exactly how the massage is done!

People will ask, "How long should I do massage? When should I stop?" Breast massage is recommended essentially forever. This might sound hard, but it is not. Once the breasts have softened, massage can be simplified. Usually it is done just once a day for a minute or two. Typically, the pinch exercise is stopped and we just do the side to side exercise. It often is done during a person's daily shower. This is a good time to do it. It is continued to minimize scar tissue formation.

Depending on your personal settling and healing, I will review and modify massage. This emphasizes the importance of follow up visits. Don't miss these. Some people might drop a bit too low. I might have these patients stop doing massage. Others might continue with the pinching on the top for longer periods or more frequently than other patients. I tailor the treatment for your own anatomy and healing.

Doing regular breast augmentation massage after surgery does not guarantee that a person will not get capsular contracture. It is done to decrease the chance of this problem.

**Shoulder Exercises and Posture:**

Because breast implants cause pain, it is common for people to assume a forward appearing or slouched posture. It's a normal splinting mechanism that the body does when it suffers pain in the chest area. This posture, however, can contribute to a higher location of the implants and can hinder the settling process.

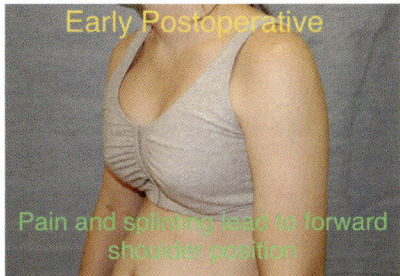 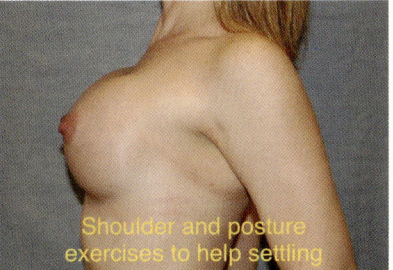

By assuming a shoulder down and shoulder back position, we can help with the settling and dropping of the implants. This exercise helps with breast massage. This exercise and posture will be described and shown to you in detail after surgery by me. By placing the shoulders down and back, it stretches the pectoralis muscle. This leads to a gradual stretching of the surrounding tissue and improvement of the appearance and location of the implants. It is done 10 times a day, and the position is held for 2 minutes.

## What if I had a breast lift too?

If a patient has breast implants and a breast lift, the instructions for the breast massage technique might be completely different to allow for better healing. It will depend on your prior hanging, shape, and healing. I will review this with you personally during your recovery. You should still read my educational writings on massage and watch the video on my web page. Please be prepared. So to repeat, if you also have a breast lift with your augmentation, breast massage might be different than a person with just implant surgery. I will review exactly what is best for you.

Chapter 12

# Breast Augmentation Settling

## Summary

After cosmetic augmentation, changes happen with the shape and the appearance of the breasts. This process happens slowly and is called settling. During this period, the tissues stretch and the implants drop. As this occurs, women will see a more natural and attractive look to their breasts.

The recovery after breast augmentation takes time as healing occurs. The implants drop and the nipple will gradually move up. There are massage techniques and shoulder exercises that can help you recover and settle. This chapter will focus on this important aspect of breast augmentation.

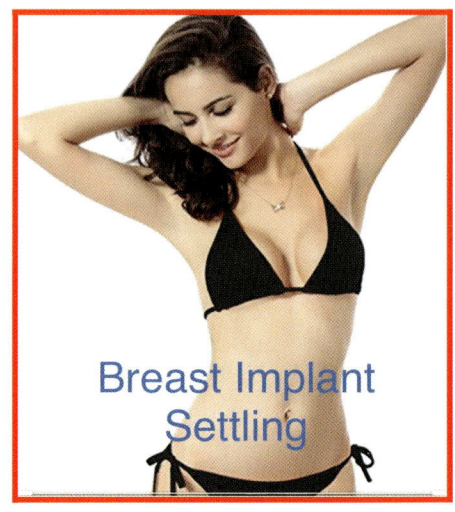

## Overview:

Cosmetic breast augmentation is one of the most commonly performed cosmetic surgery procedures done each year. Statistics by the American Society of Plastic Surgery usually show that this operation is in the top 3 done every year. Results and patient satisfaction are very high with the operation.

However, women need to understand that it is not an operation where the breast implants are placed and *presto-chango* you wake up with perfect breasts. It takes time for healing to occur, and this is what the chapter will focus on. Breast augmentation involves putting breast implants behind the muscle. They are almost always placed in this location. The predominant muscle is the pectoralis major muscle but also the serratis anterior on the side to a lesser degree.

The placement of breast implants behind the muscle is called submuscular breast augmentation. The muscle provides *soft tissue* coverage and improved results. The muscle helps give a softer and more natural result with lower risks. However, the space behind the muscle is very tight at first, and it takes time for this space to stretch out.

This process or stretching is commonly referred to as dropping, settling, and/or drop and fluff. These are layman terms for settling and the changes that occur after this cosmetic breast operation. This stretching out of the muscle does take time. Usually it is a short period of time, but sometimes several months or even longer is necessary. Most people, however, can look good in just a couple of weeks. This is true especially in clothing or swim suits, but undressed it can take longer to look completely natural, as you settle and heal.

## How Long Does It Take?

This process of settling of breast implants is gradual as just described. It does take time for the muscles to stretch out and relax. It is similar to the slow changes that happen to the abdominal muscles with pregnancy. Human tissues take time to stretch out during recovery. Your breast and muscle need time to settle.

In my experience, the vast majority of settling occurs in the first month. Additional settling happens over the next 2 months. Some people can require longer to heal and drop completely. Classically, it's all done at 6 months, although some doctors will say 1 year.

**Change in Appearance:**

During this process of settling, the breasts will gradually change and soften. The shape and appearance changes also. The breasts tend to slowly look less round and more natural. It takes time, so be patient. Sometimes the breasts even look bigger as the muscle relaxes and the implants *come out.*

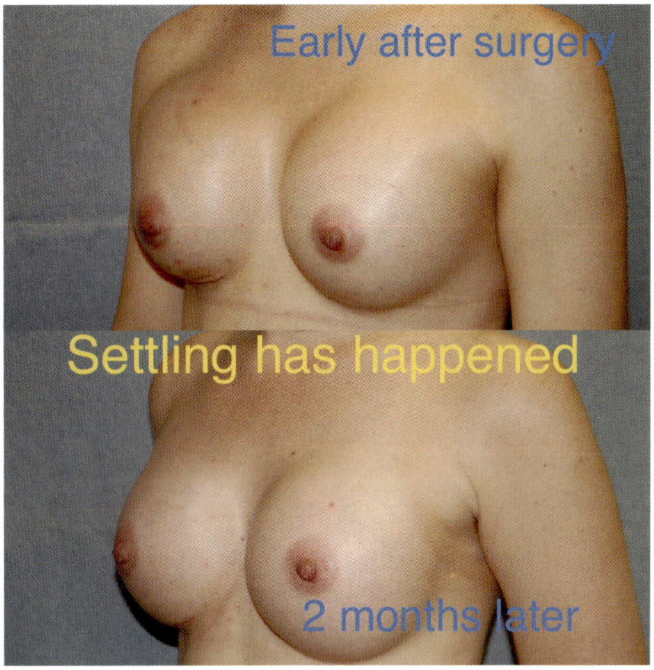

The nipple location varies with the position of the implant. This is important because woman can worry about the nipples appearing at first too low. As breast enlargement settling gradually occurs and the implants *drop*, the nipple position appears to change. When the implant drops, the nipple appears to go up. It might seem unusual, but breast implant settling or breast implant dropping occurs inside. So as the breast implant drops, the nipple moves up. This is extremely normal and common. The picture to the right demonstrates this.

**Two Phases:**

Breast augmentation recovery can be viewed as having two phases. The first phase is the short period around the actual operation. This is the part, unfortunately, where pain is involved. However, I use a Pain Buster to really decrease this pain and help make it as pain free as possible. The second phase of breast augmentation recovery is this slow stretching of the tissue and muscle that is called breast dropping or settling.

This second phase does take time as described above, but usually there is no real pain with this phase. Breast massage or implant displacement are stretching maneuvers that are done to speed up the breast implant dropping. I have a video that shows this in detail, and you can see this on my webpage at ChrisSaundersMD.Com. Massage techniques and posture exercises will help speed up the settling process. This is reviewed in Chapter 10. Women are encouraged to review this chapter and to focus on the massage techniques. This will help you settle. By doing this, you will stretch out the tissues and look and feel better more quickly.

Chapter 13

# Tummy Tuck

## Summary

A tummy tuck or an abdominoplasty is a wonderful operation designed to make the stomach area flatter, thinner, and more sculpted. This procedure can give patients a flat stomach area that they have only dreamed about. I have personally been amazed at the results, and I believe the satisfaction of this operation is one of the best in cosmetic surgery. Women will say, can push up my breasts in a bra, but I can't do anything with this stomach." It also can be combined with breast surgery and is called a *Mommy Makeover*.

However, it is important to understand the recovery from this operation. Because it involves muscle tightening, the pain is more than most operations. The Pain Buster has dramatically reduced this pain, and I believe it has revolutionized this recovery. But nevertheless, pain is a big part of this operation for the first several days. It's best to be honest and be prepared mentally for this aspect of the surgery. Please read Chapter 7 on the Pain Buster. It is an amazing machine that can help you.

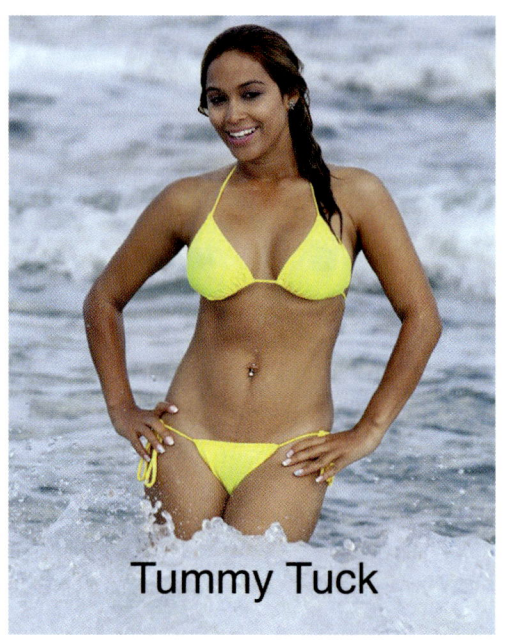

"I

**Tummy Tuck**

The tummy tuck is an abdominal operation with moderate risk of blood clots. I emphasize this risk as probably the single greatest thing to focus on after surgery. We do not want a blood clot. The chapter on DVT and blood clots and their prevention is mandatory reading. As with all operations, it is extremely important to follow instructions closely. This chapter will outline the specific instructions that I recommend to heal the best from a tummy tuck operation.

Finally, as with all operations, please refrain from smoking, nicotine patches, or nicotine gum. Nicotine can seriously affect the outcome of tummy tuck surgery. Even secondhand smoke can contribute to increased complications. This is emphasized because of its extreme importance. Nicotine can diminish blood supply to the healing incision and lead to complications and scarring that can be extremely severe. The instruction to *do not smoke* is an absolute mandatory warning that must that be taken extremely seriously.

## Overnight stay:

Tummy tucks are one of the operations where I recommend an overnight stay. Typically, this is done in the hotel that is 1 block from my deluxe surgery center. Please see Chapter 9 on the surgery center and its advantages. The overnight stay in the hotel includes private duty nursing care with a one on one ratio. This allows for the best nursing care in my opinion. It leads to excellent education of instructions to the patient and also diminished anxiety and fear. I come to you and do a postoperative check the next morning to assess how you are doing. Patients typically go home in the morning to continue recovery with family and/or friends assisting at home.

**Bandages:**

It is normal to have bloody bandages after an abdominoplasty. Most of this will occur the night of surgery and will gradually diminish over the next several days. In general, the bandages are not changed unless they are excessively bloody. They are placed at surgery and are sterile. I believe it minimizes infection to leave them alone if bleeding is minimal, as is typically the case. In the situation where we have more than a little bleeding, the bandages are changed or reinforced. Reinforcing means placing additional gauze on top of the old gauze. Hands should be washed or gloves worn. Do not touch the incision or where the drains come out the skin. Classically, this is addressed by me the following day after surgery during your postoperative check. After you have showered, it is ok to not have the incision covered by gauze. It is ok, however, to replace gauze on the incision, if this makes you feel comfortable. Otherwise a T-shirt is worn to provide padding for the incision, and then the abdominal binder is replaced on top of the T-shirt. Drains are secured via pins to the abdominal binder. Chapter 14 covers drains and their management in detail. Photos in this chapter will help you see how to cover the incision and manage the drains.

**Drains:**

Drains are unfortunately necessary after an abdominoplasty. I believe that if drains are not used, you ultimately will have more fluid, swelling, and blood accumulation. I believe that doctors who *do not* use drains will *not* get the best results and as flat a stomach as when drains are routinely used. The drains stay in approximately 1 week. They are a nuisance, but they are very manageable. They give us the best results, and help us heal. Drains can be messy, and this should be considered as normal. It is very common to have drainage around the tubes, and this can be discomforting. It is ok to place gauze around where the tube exits the skin. As discussed, do not touch where the tube exits the skin.

The nurses will teach you how to empty and record the drains. It is actually not difficult, and do not fear this. This is best done between 8 to 9 o'clock in the morning and a second time between 8 and 9 o'clock in the evening. Initially after surgery, it might have to be emptied 3 or 4 times instead of just twice a day. Record the output from the drains on a piece of paper, so this can be followed by me during the recovery period. The metric system is printed on the side of the JP drain. This will allow you to precisely measure how much is coming out in ml's.

After emptying the drain, it is important to re-squeeze the drain, because this is how it applies suction. If the drain bulb is open and not compressed, it does not give suction to the system.
*Chapter 13 is mandatory reading and reviews this in detail*.

**Pain Pump or Pain Buster:**

The Pain Pump or the Pain Buster is a machine that delivers medication continuously to the surgical site for 3 days. I believe it has revolutionized the recovery from a tummy tuck. The days of overnight stays in a hospital with intravenous narcotic medication are long gone. The medicine inside the Pain Buster is lidocaine. This is the medicine used by dentists to numb your gums. The machine is in a fanny pack around your waist. It delivers a continuous supply of lidocaine to the tummy tuck surgical site to diminish pain.

Because it is filled with lidocaine, the pain pump is completely safe and is not a morphine ball. The medicine or lidocaine is so safe, you can actually drink it. Although this is not what its purpose is for. The pain pump lasts 3 days and this is usually long enough to get you through the worst part of the recovery. Most people have significantly less pain by 3 days and do well with just oral medication.

The pain pump is not adjustable, however, so you cannot turn it up or turn it down. It is also common to have some of the medication leak out of the system around the tube, so this area can become wet. This is of no concern, and do not worry.

The pain pump is meant to be removed by the patient. This is done 3 days after surgery. It should be removed at the same time as the first shower, which is approximately 72 hours after surgery. The pain pump can be discarded at this point and does not need to be returned to the office.

**Blood Clot and DVT Prevention:**

It is extremely important to understand blood clots and their relationship with abdominal surgery. Blood clot and DVT are synonymous and imply the same thing. DVT means deep venous thrombosis (clot). The prevention of blood clots cannot be over emphasized. An interesting fact is that there are approximately 100,000 blood clot deaths each year in America. This is more deaths than from car accidents and breast cancer combined. It is this important fact that makes it imperative that we understand the best way to minimize and to try and prevent blood clots.

Blood clots can happen after any surgical procedure, but it has an increased risk with tummy tucks. it is because of this fact that I take special effort and precautions to make risks as low as possible. There are 4 things we do to minimize this complication. The first is *early ambulation*. This means getting up and walking around the house for approximately 10 minutes 10 times a day. This has been shown to diminish blood clot risks. The second thing I recommend is *leg compression stockings.* A common brand is Jobst. The compression stockings squeeze the veins and keep or minimize blood from accumulating in them.

The third factor I recommend is to *keep the legs elevated* above the heart. I call it the "tilted back lounge chair" position. If the legs are above the heart, then blood dependently drains through gravity. The final factor is what I call *the invisible bicycle.* This is a recommendation to pump and move the legs almost continuously during the postoperative period. I have had excellent success when patients follow these 4 recommended prevention methods. Blood clot risks are elevated for approximately 1 month after surgery. These instructions should be followed for 1 month after your tummy tuck. *Chapter 5 which is devoted to blood clots and their prevention is mandatory reading.*

**Showering:**

Your first shower is 72 hours or 3 days after the completion of your surgery. This allows enough time for the incision to seal and it is safe to shower at this point. You are allowed to shower, but not to soak in a bath or a hot tub. These would be major mistakes. At the shower, the pain pump and urinary catheter are removed. After these are removed, you should be left with just the drainage tubes. For the shower, use mild soap and water. Do not remove the Steri-Strips. These are left on 1 week. It is wise to have a sitting stool present at the shower, because it is not uncommon to feel lightheaded at this first shower. It is also recommended that you have someone help you for the shower.

After the shower, bandages are no longer necessary for the incision. A cotton T-shirt is recommended to provide padding and comfort beneath the binder or girdle. Gauze can be reapplied for comfort and extra padding if desired. The binder is reapplied on top of the T-shirt. The drains are then re-fastened to the binder to make sure they are secure and do not get accidentally pulled out.

**Activity:**

Please see Chapter 5 on blood clot prevention. The invisible bicycle should be done almost continuously when you are in bed. When you are walking after a tummy tuck, please walk slightly bent over at the waist to take tension off of the incision. *No twisting* or rotating of the waist or trunk is recommended. Twisting can hinder healing and lead to increased fluid production. For the first couple of weeks after the surgery, we are predominantly walking around the house as our main activity. As we heal and the drainage tubes are successfully removed, I will recommend increased activity.

As I have emphasized above, twisting at the waist can lead to the skin moving back-and-forth over the muscle repair and can lead to increased risks and fluid production. Try and wear the binder at all times, and try not to twist at the waist. This promotes healthy healing.

If things are going well, I recommend increased activity from weeks 2 to 6 after the surgery. I call this the *phased-in* activity period. During this period, a patient might be able to resume light household activities, driving, and work. Some activities like a stationary bicycle in the gym or an elliptical (while holding on) would be acceptable, if healing is going well. I will give you the ok when you can proceed with these increased activities. After 6 weeks, unlimited activity is ok, if I have approved it.

**Binder and Garments:**

And abdominal binder is provided as part of the tummy tuck for you to wear after surgery. Sometimes this is a more extensive compression garment if liposuction of the thighs and legs have been done. At the time of the first shower, the binder or garment can be washed and dried. You can be in a bathrobe until the washing cycle is complete. The binder is white, so it's not uncommon for it to get stained. You can hit this garment hard with bleach to get it extra clean.

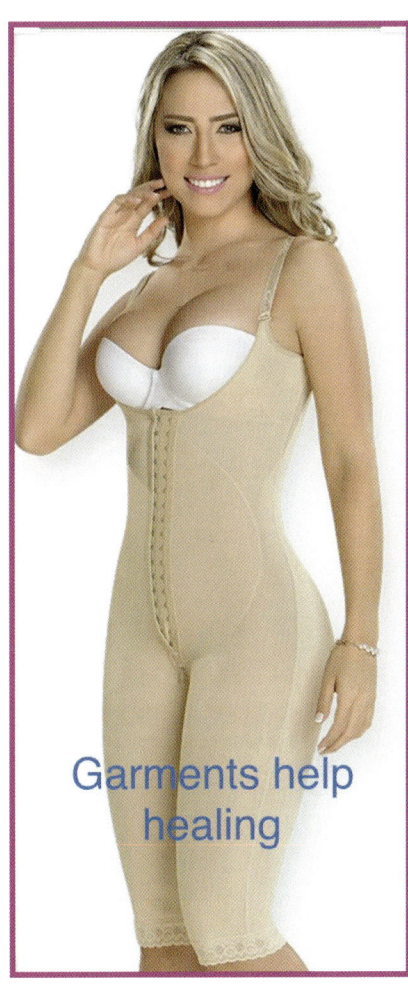

Garments help healing

Initially the binder should not be too tight. It should be loosely applied to hold gauze over the incision and to allow for securing of the drainage tubes. As you heal, I will recommend that the binder become increasingly tight, and this will be reviewed with you. It should not be applied too tight initially, as it could cause injury.

**Urinary Catheter:**

The urinary catheter or Foley catheter is placed at the time of surgery. It is placed to decompress the bladder and to monitor your urine output. I leave the urinary catheter in for approximately 72 hours and recommend removal at your first shower. Some doctors will recommend removal earlier, but I have found that by leaving it in several days it gives extra ability to monitor how well you physiologically are doing. It also can be safely removed comfortably at the shower. Risks are extremely low with the catheter.

## Ambulation:

As discussed above, it is important to get up and move around after an abdominoplasty. This is called early ambulation medically. It is wise to have assistance during the initial several days after surgery. I call this *out of bed with assistance*. This is because it's common to feel lightheaded, and people can fall. If a loved one or helper is there to give a helping hand or support, it diminishes the chances of a fall or accident. As you heal, feeling lightheaded and fainting becomes much less common, and most people can then get out of bed and walk about without assistance.

Initially after this operation, when you go from a lying down to a sitting position, go slowly so you do not feel excessively lightheaded. When you go from sitting to standing, go slowly again so we don't faint. Medically these are called transfers. Transfers mean changing from one position to another. Go slow with all transfers after surgery. This means go slow from lying down to sitting and then go slow again when going from sitting to standing.

## Medications:

It is required to take all of the antibiotics prescribed by me. Intravenous antibiotics are given before surgery. Start your oral antibiotic when you go home. The other medications for pain, nausea, and anxiety are optional. Most people will need some supplementary pain medication as the pain pump is fantastic, but it does not give you zero pain.

In addition to the narcotic medication, I allow patients to take Tylenol or Motrin to supplement with their pain control. 4 Motrin tablets at a time give excellent pain relief for most patients. The maximum Motrin is 12 tablets a day.

The anxiety medicine or Valium is also a muscle relaxant. It can provide additional comfort by diminishing muscle spasms associated with the tightening of muscles during a tummy tuck. This can be safely taken with the pain pills or staggered. Staggered means taking the two medications and alternating them every 2 hours.

Chapter 14

# Tummy Tuck Recovery - Drains, Care, and Underwear

## Summary

This chapter covers how to care for your drains. It also reviews what you can expect and what underwear and clothing is best after your tummy tuck or abdominoplasty operation. It is important to be educated and to understand the drains and their care.

Abdominoplasty surgery can make fabulous improvement to the stomach area making it flatter, thinner, and more sculpted. Recovery does take time however, and patients need to be ready and educated for this phase of the operation. Drainage tubes are necessary to collect fluid after the operation. The great majority of doctors use drainage tubes, because they believe it gives better results with lower risks. Some doctors don't use them, but I believe this is not wise. I also believe you will *not get* as flat a stomach if they are not used. I believe they are a critical part of the healing process. They are a temporary nuisance, but they will lead to the flattest stomach and the best results.

The drains are plastic *balls* or *bulbs* that work by suction. They are classically called Jackson-Pratt (JP) drains. This is a brand. The drain ball is connected to a tube that is placed at the time of surgery. At the end of the tube there are a lot of holes that suck up fluid. The fluid is called serous fluid. This is bloody tinged fluid. The fluid will sometimes have blood clots in them. This is ok. It is not the blood clots that form in the legs that are of serious concern. The drainage ball *must be squeezed flat.* This creates the suction to suck out the fluid. It doesn't work if it is not squeezed.

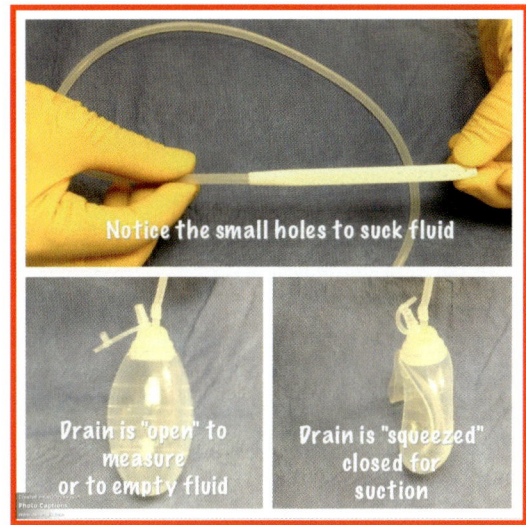

Notice the small holes to suck fluid

Drain is "open" to measure or to empty fluid

Drain is "squeezed" closed for suction

Tummy tuck drain care is very easy. Clean your hands before and after touching them. Hands have bacteria on them, and hand washing decreases bacteria and the chance of infection. Also, don't touch the tube where the tube goes in the skin. This can increase your chance of causing infection or a problem. Use a Q-tip or gloved hand to apply Neosporin, Bacitracin, or Triple Antibiotic ointment once or twice a day to where the tube enters the skin. After the ointment is applied, cover the first part of the tube with gauze or panty liners. It doesn't have to be sterile, but clean gauze or panty liners is fine. This is for hygiene purposes too. Daily showers are also recommended as this keeps the area clean and minimizes infection.

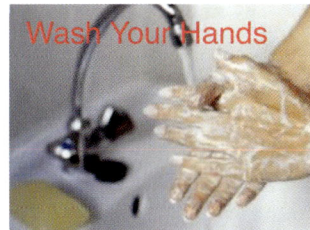

Wash Your Hands

Empty and record drainage amount from the drain twice a day. The first few days after surgery you might have to empty it more frequently. Empty them extra times if the ball gets too full. This will minimize the chance of spillage or making a mess. There are numbers on the side of the drainage ball. These numbers are ml's or cc's. These are equivalent and are used for the measurements. Do the measuring when the ball is open or not squeezed. You should write down these numbers.

The fluid can then get discarded in the sink or toilet. The amount of fluid draining will determine when the tubes are removed. Expect the number to gradually decrease. Sometimes it will drain less and other days more. It is common for this to go up and down. The trend tends to be less with time. The first several days you might have to empty it more than twice a day.

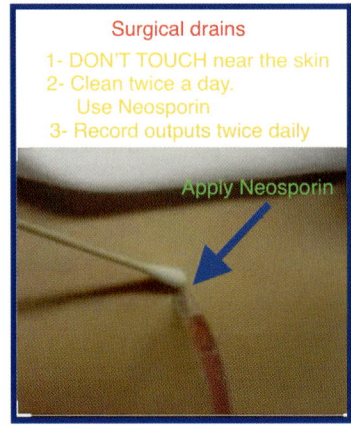

Surgical drains
1- DON'T TOUCH near the skin
2- Clean twice a day.
Use Neosporin
3- Record outputs twice daily

Apply Neosporin

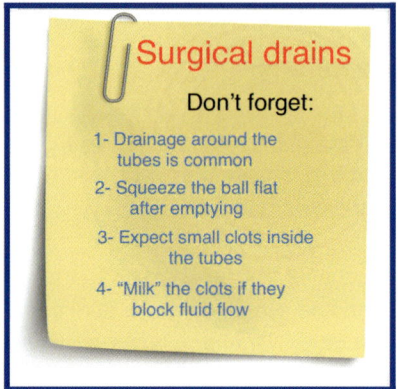

Surgical drains
Don't forget:
1- Drainage around the tubes is common
2- Squeeze the ball flat after emptying
3- Expect small clots inside the tubes
4- "Milk" the clots if they block fluid flow

As mentioned above, it is common for small blood clots to get in the tubes. These are not the blood clots known as DVT or Deep Venous Thrombosis. These small clots in the tube have nothing to do with those clots. These are just part of the healing after the tummy tuck. However, the small clots can clog up the drains. This might require *milking* or *stripping* the tube. This means you slowly push the clot along the tube, so the clot gradually goes in the ball. The nurse or I will show you how it is done. It sounds scary, but is very easy.

The tube is pinched with one hand to hold it steady. With the second hand, two fingers are used to gently pinch and slowly advance the blood clot forward. Do it several times. This will gradually lead to clearing of the tube.

I recommend wearing underwear over the drain and groin area. Certain styles are best. Thongs or no underwear are not recommended. Wear older styles like *granny panties* or *boy-shorts*. These are also called "full coverage cottons." The fabrics and color do not matter. Make sure the drain comes down where the leg comes out. Don't have it come out over the top. After the underwear is on, I recommend you use a cotton T-shirt. This must be long enough to cover the groin area. It should not stop short at the pubic hair line. We want it to completely cover the entire area. It provides extra soft padding for the incision and the healing process. Finally, the abdominal binder is placed. The drains are fastened to the binder.

Drainage tubes stay in about 7-10 days.  It is very common to have drainage around the tube. This means the fluid can run down your leg. This can be concerning or worrisome, but it is normal and to be expected. The drainage tubes collect most of the fluid, but not all of it. The gauze or panty liners will collect the extra fluid. If this happens too much, look to see if a clot is blocking the tube. This can be *milked forward* as described above to help the tubes work. Each visit to the office will allow my nurses and me to check your healing and drainage tubes. They may sound scary, but most people find they are not really all that bad. I believe they are extremely important. I also find they can help us get the extra flat stomach we want after an abdominoplasty or tummy tuck!

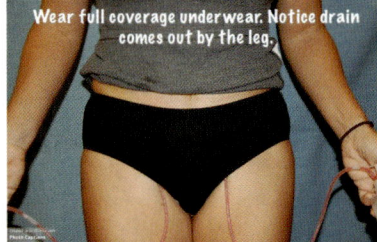

Wear full coverage underwear. Notice drain comes out by the leg.

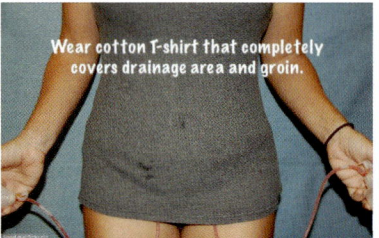

Wear cotton T-shirt that completely covers drainage area and groin.

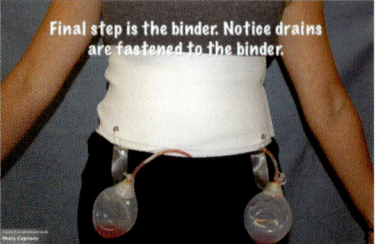

Final step is the binder. Notice drains are fastened to the binder.

Chapter 15

# Facelift and Neck Lift

## Summary

Facelift and neck lift procedures are done to rejuvenate the face including the cheeks, jaw line, jowls, and including the neck area. These operations are extremely effective in making us look younger, healthy, and youthful. Success rates are extremely high with very low risks for the majority of patients. The incisions are placed in privileged locations around the ears and are tucked behind the tragus of the ear. This location allows for incisions that fade better than any other part of the body. Chapter 6 on *Incisions and Scars* reviews this topic in detail. The recovery is characterized by very little pain but significant bruising. It takes time for the bruising to resolve. I describe it as a hibernation period, where you are home resting and letting the bruising go away.

It is critically important to understand that you must relax and take it easy after facial procedures. Some people have said, "Doc, I know I have to rest and chill out." This is their way of describing the importance of resting and relaxing after a facelift. It is described below and is paramount to review.

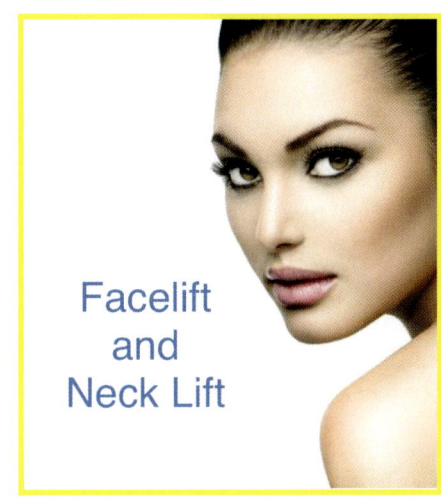

Facelift
and
Neck Lift

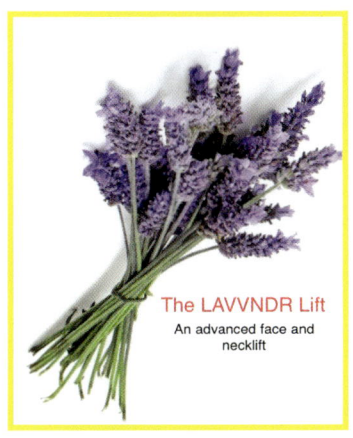

The LAVVNDR Lift
An advanced face and
necklift

This operation has a distinctly different recovery than operations like a tummy tuck or breast augmentation. I'll describe it as having a different *flavor*. Facelifts tend to have very little pain. It can be surprising how little pain there is for many people. However, they have visible bruising that needs to resolve before you can get back to your normal life. Tummy tucks and breast augmentation have the opposite recovery with much more pain and no visible bruising. To repeat myself, facial operations tend to have very little pain but visible bruising, since it's on the face. It will take time for the bruising to resolve. I think this is excellent news for most patients. The pain is minimal for most. We just have to allow time and *hibernation to heal.*

I specialize in these operations. The LAVVNDR Lift as shown in the picture is my personally created operation. As with all cosmetic surgery procedures, it is important to have realistic expectations about how young these operations make us look. They do not turn a person into a movie star or into a 25 year old person. These operations ONLY help us and ONLY improve us. Understand they have limitations in how young you will actually look. This chapter describes the recovery from these wonderful cosmetic facial operations.

## Head Elevation:

It is important to keep your head elevated at all times. This includes sleeping. This can be done in a lounge chair or in a bed with multiple pillows. Please maintain at least a 45° angle of head elevation. The head elevation minimizes bruising, swelling, and problems with healing. As with all instructions, this is extremely important and your head should not be put down for one second.

Think about what happens when you put your head down to tie your shoes. When I do this, blood rushes to my head, and my head turns red. If this was done shortly after surgery, the blood rushing down to the face can actually start up bleeding and increase bruising and swelling. It is something we do not want to do at all. *It is extremely important to keep your head elevated at all times, including when sleeping.* Head elevation should be for approximately 2 weeks. It is absolutely critical during the first 3 to 5 days. I will let you know based upon healing when this becomes less important.

**Chin Up:**

*Chin up* means that the chin area is extended up and away from your chest. If you are at a 45° inclination with your head elevated, the chin up position would mean that your face is looking up to the ceiling. This chin up position takes tension off of the incisions and increases the blood supply to the areas that are healing. I have found this to be extremely important and should be followed strictly until further notice, usually 3 to 5 days.

Reading is a chin down position. Recovering from a facelift can be boring and so reading is something that is often done. It's something that I would do after surgery. However, the book needs to be elevated so you can maintain the chin up position. Neck rolls or airplane pillows can assist you in getting the chin up and maintaining the chin up position. No pressure on the front of the neck is allowed. So, no rolls or pillows on the front of the neck.

It's ok to put your chin down to walk or go to the bathroom. It's also ok to put your chin down to eat at the kitchen table for a short period of time. Most of the time the chin should be continuously elevated until further notice. This instruction for the strict chin elevation is usually for the first 3 to 5 days. After your healing, it becomes less important, and I will instruct you when you can assume a more neutral or natural position of your neck.

**Rest, Relax, and Whisper:**

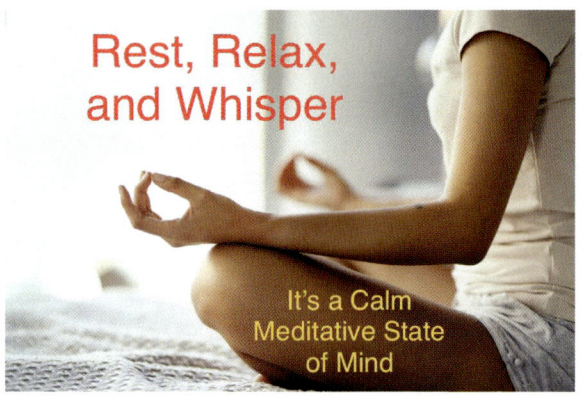

This is a concept. It is extremely important. It's one that I think people have the hardest time following after surgery. *It means after surgery that we need to be relaxed with low anxiety and low blood pressure.* It's good to be in a meditative mindset, relaxed, whispering, and calm. I am going to explain why this is extremely important.

In medicine there is a term called a Valsalva. It's when we bear down and contract our core muscles. The bearing down might be to lift heavy objects or to have a bowel movement. When a person bears down or has a Valsalva, the body contracts and the diaphragm contracts and sends blood up through the jugular venous system into our head. Just like when we lift a heavy object, our face might turn red. Valsalvas are a big problem after cosmetic facial surgery. Imagine someone screaming and yelling after surgery. Their face would turn red, and they could increase bleeding and hinder healing. They could actual start bleeding! Screaming is a big valsalva. But here is something that is interesting. Laughing is also a Valsalva. So we don't do yelling or screaming, but we also don't do laughing after surgery. Even loud talking is a form of Valsalva. Imagine the orator in a big lecture hall, as he talks, the veins in his face stand out as he uses small valsalva contractions of his diaphragm to project his voice. So the *rest, relax, and whisper* is understanding that after surgery, we are lying down, relaxed, calm, and almost in a meditative state. There's no laughing, screaming, yelling, bearing down, talking loud, lifting, or high anxiety. We also try to not throw up, strain at bowel movements, cough, or sneeze. Some of these things are impossible not to do after surgery, and this is understood. But we do our best to minimize all these activities. The wise patient will literally whisper, "I understand you Dr. Saunders; I'm just going to sit here quietly, calmly, and heal as best I can!"

I prescribe anxiety medications to all my patients. Some people will need them after these operations to help relax. This is good to do. If you know your personality is on the high anxiety side, then be prepared to use this medication to help relax and recover.

## Bruising and Swelling:

Facial operations will have significant bruising and swelling. This is normal and to be expected. The bruising will also travel down because of gravity. So, it is more visible in the neck and sometimes even the upper chest area. This is called dependent drainage. The bruising and swelling are at its peak 1or 2 days after surgery. The more ice and elevation you do, the quicker this will resolve. The majority of the bruising goes away over 10-14 days. I will tell patients that 10 days after surgery, you are cleared to go out to dinner with a loved one. You are medically cleared. However, you may have residual bruising that you wish to hide. If this is of concern, then it can be hidden with make-up. Some patients will want more time to allow the extra bruising to go away. Allow 4 to 6 weeks before big functions or weddings to feel the most comfortable. Think of the recovery from bruising as like a hibernation period. You just need to give it time to allow for it to go away.

## Icing:

Ice application to the cheeks, face, and neck area is good after surgery. It's extremely important for the first 72 hours. No direct ice application to the skin. The crushed ice should be placed in a Ziploc bag and covered by a damp washcloth to avoid direct contact of the ice to the skin. Reusable ice packs are good too, but please cover them with a damp washcloth to avoid direct skin contact. I recommend icing to be done approximately 20 minutes on and 20 minutes off, whenever you are awake.

## Bandages:

The bandage goes around the head and the neck area. Your eyes, nose, and mouth are purposely not covered. Try not to disrupt the bandage, as it has been meticulously placed by me after surgery. If it does become disrupted by accident, please re-wrap it, but keep it on the loose side. A tight bandage could cause injury.

There's a mandatory visit in the office the next day after surgery. The bandage will be changed for a clean one. It tends to be much more comfortable. This is when you get to see your face for the first time after surgery. So the first visit is a fun one, as you get to see the beginning of the healing process and see your new face.

This bandage is worn for 72 hours at which point it can be discarded. This happens to be also the time that you're allowed to shower for the first time.

**Bleeding:**

It's common to have some spotting of blood around and behind the ears on the first bandage. This is normal. It will be changed on your first visit, which is the day after surgery. As per the general instructions, please call if you believe you have excessive bleeding. This is not common, however. Some blood is to be expected after all operations.

**Showering:**

You will be told when to shower afterwards, which is approximately 72 hours or 3 days after surgery. At this time you can wash your face and hair with shampoo. Please be gentle, and don't pull at any sutures or clips that have been used for the operation. Please let your hair air dry, and do not use a hair dryer until after 7 to 10 days.

**Medications:**

It is imperative to take the antibiotics that were prescribed by me. Pain medication, nausea medication, and anxiety medication are also prescribed and to are be used as needed. The anxiety medicine might help some people rest, relax, and whisper that was discussed above. Be careful about the pain medication. Narcotics can make some people throw up, and we don't want this. Tylenol and Motrin usually are enough for most people to relieve pain.

**Incisions:**

Sutures and clips are gradually removed over approximately 5 to 10 days. They are not removed all at once for most people. If you have scabbing covering up a suture, it can hurt to remove the suture and scab at that first time. I have found it's completely safe to just let the scab gently come off and remove the suture at the next visit. This does not change the the cosmetic appearance of the incision at all. So to repeat, the sutures come out in 2 or 3 stages. Approximately a week after surgery, the vast majority of your sutures are removed. And the few remaining are removed in the subsequent week. The incision should be treated with Neosporin twice a day for 3 days and then Bio-Oil twice a day for a month.

**Exercise and Activity:**

Activity should be kept to a minimum initially. It's still important to have early ambulation and walk around the house to minimize the risk of blood clots. For the first week, we are predominately at home, allowing for bruising and swelling to resolve. We are hiding, hibernating, and relaxing. Most people can return to work after 1 week to 2 weeks. A lot of this depends on how much privacy you want. Recovering from a facelift involves a certain amount of hibernation to let bruising and swelling go away. The person who doesn't care about visible bruising and swelling can just cover it with make-up; they can go back to work after approximately 1 week. This of course depends upon your follow up visits and me approving your return to work.

Other people will need more time to allow for bruising and swelling to go away. For people who want to be extremely confidential, 2 - 4 weeks might be preferred by them. I often describe recovering from a facelift in the following way. Approximately 10 days after surgery, you and a husband or loved one can go out for dinner wearing a little bit of make-up. You will be medically cleared to go out for dinner. However, some people might have residual bruising, and if this is of concern to you, then you will need a bit more time to allow for bruising to go away. This typically means an extra week for resolution of bruising and swelling.

Chapter 16

# Eyelid Surgery or Blepharoplasty

## Summary

Eyelid lifts are also called eye tucks and medically a blepharoplasty. These are operations designed to rejuvenate and enhance the appearance of the eyelid area. In the upper eyelids, extra skin is classically called hooding. Surgery is performed to improve and rejuvenate this problem. In the lower eyelid area, the operations are done to improve bags and circles. Since we look at each other in the eyes, these operations can give dramatic amounts of rejuvenation. I personally have had his operation done and could not be more pleased. *My brother did an excellent job with my surgery, and I recommend him highly to many patients.*

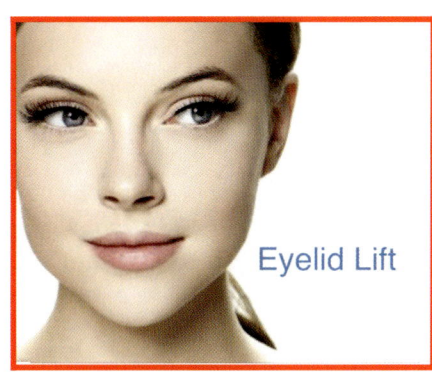

Eyelid Lift

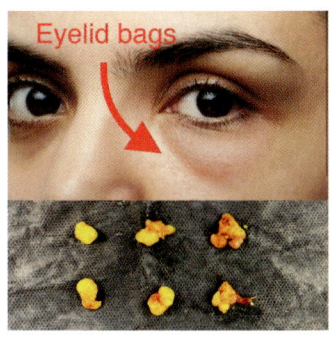

Eyelid bags

Like facelift and neck lift operations, the blepharoplasty is characterized by very little pain during recovery, but significant bruising. Even plastic surgery text books will say that if someone is having a lot of pain, than something is wrong. Most people have very little pain. I didn't even take a Tylenol, when I had my operation done. But bruising is around the eyes. So people will see it. This takes time to resolve.

The eyes are the first place that facial aging occurs for many. Since we look at each other in the eyes, this is a good place to start for those wanting to look younger. Extra skin around the eyes and eyelid bags are the main reasons we look tired and old in the eyes. The picture on the left shows actual eyelid bags removed by me at surgery. It is also much less expensive than facelift operations. Many plastic surgeons consider the eye tuck to be one of the best operations we do. This is because the operation is highly successful, has extremely low risks, has high satisfaction rates, and is very reasonable in cost.

## Head Elevation:

Strict head elevation is extremely important. Strict means that this it is done at all times with no exceptions. This includes sleeping at night. It should be at least 45° of elevation. Do not let your head come down for even a second, as this can increase bruising, swelling, and the chance of bleeding.

## Rest, Relax, and Whisper:

This was described in detail in the facelift chapter. The concept is the same. After eyelid surgery, it's extremely important to be in a calm, relaxed, and stress-free atmosphere. Rest, relax, and whisper is a concept. It's an idea that we need to calmly rest to allow for the best healing. Valsalva is the medical word for any type of bearing down. This includes yelling, screaming, but also it includes things like laughing or talking. During a Valsalva, we bear down and the diaphragm contracts. The blood is shunted up the jugular system to our head and can increase bleeding and delay healing. We want to avoid all activities that do this.

This means that we avoid laughing, yelling, screaming, and talking. That's why you are told to whisper. But, it also means we try to avoid things such as throwing up, sneezing, and coughing. Some things like throwing up cannot be avoided, however, we try our best not to. We also want to be low anxiety and calm. Try and be in a meditative state of mind. Try and maintain this calm and relaxed attitude to heal well.

Rest, relax, and whisper is extremely important after eyelid surgery. It cannot be over emphasized. It is critically important for the first 3 to 5 days, and if we are healing well these restrictions are taken away in a short period of time.

## Bleeding:

It's normal to have some drops of blood from the eyelid incision. It's not a lot of blood, but sometimes you will have a tiny trickle of blood running down your cheek. You can't bandage the eyes, so it is common to have some minor amount of blood come out. It will drip out or get on the washcloth when icing. Ice application is described below. The bleeding is very minimal and usually stops within the first 1 or 2 days.

## Bruising and Swelling:

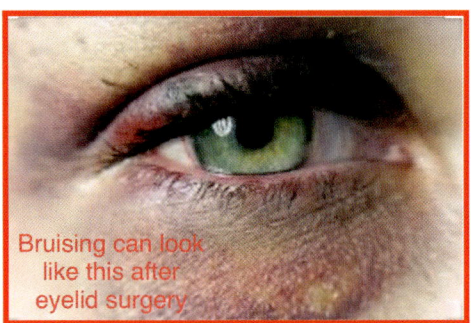

Bruising can look like this after eyelid surgery

Facial operations will have significant bruising and swelling. This is normal and to be expected. The bruising will also travel down because of gravity. So, it is more visible in the lower eyes and sometimes cheeks. This is called dependent drainage. The bruising and swelling are at its peak 1 or 2 days after surgery. The more ice and elevation you do, the quicker this will resolve. The majority of the bruising goes away over 10-14 days. I will tell patients that 10 days after surgery, you are cleared to go out to dinner with a loved one. You are medically cleared. However, you may have residual bruising that you wish to hide. If this is of concern, then it can be hidden with make-up. Some patients will want more time to allow the extra bruising to go away. Allow 4 to 6 weeks before big functions or weddings to feel the most comfortable. Think of the bruising as needing a hibernation period. You just need to give it time to allow for it to go away.

## Eyes Closed:

The eyes heal best when they are closed. This is extremely important. The eyes can have delayed healing, if they are open too much. We live in a modern world with cell phones, computers, and TVs. Too much screen time will dry out the eyes and hinder healing. *It's extremely important to keep the eyes closed almost continuously for the first 3 to 5 days after surgery.*

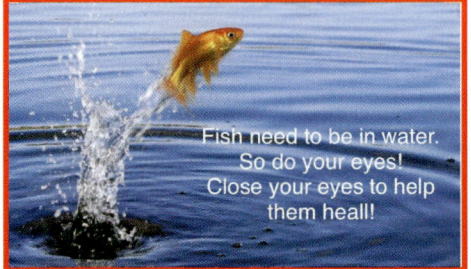

Fish need to be in water. So do your eyes! Close your eyes to help them heal!

The eyes are like fish. Fish need to be in water to live. We put our eyes in water by closing them. This allows for the eyes to be bathed in our natural tears. Tears have oxygen and give the cornea and eye the oxygen necessary for healing. If the eyes are kept open, the eyes will dry out and become injected and red. Think of it like a fish flopping on the deck of a boat, the fish needs to be put back in the water quickly. To get your eyes to heal well, you need to close them to get them in the water. It sounds so simple, but I can't over emphasize this key feature.

## Icing of the Eyes:

In addition to being closed, the eyes should be iced. This is recommended almost continuously for the first 3 to 5 days. After appropriate healing, we can slow down on the icing. The way I like you to ice your eyes is with crushed ice in a Ziploc bag. Cover the bag with a moist washcloth that has been dipped in ice cold water. The crushed ice in a Ziplock bag can be replaced by a refreezable or reusable ice bag. No frozen peas or steaks are allowed, as this is not hygienic.

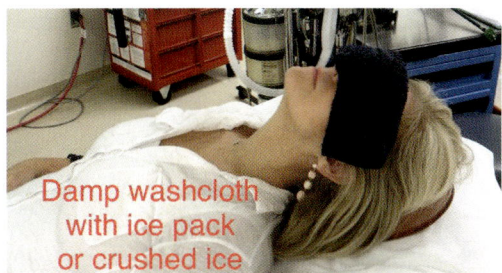

Damp washcloth with ice pack or crushed ice

The ice bag also applies a small amount of pressure to the eyelid area, and this is good for the healing process. Sometimes the ice bags can be wrapped around your head to secure them. They should be snug, but not tight. It should be wrapped just enough to hold them in place.

## Showering:

Showering is allowed the day after surgery. Please do not get soap or shampoo in the eyes. The face can be cleansed with a washcloth and mild soak.

## Medications:

The antibiotics are mandatory to take after surgery and are started when you get home. If your stomach is upset, you can start them the next day. Intravenous antibiotics are given to you prior to your operation. The pain medication, anxiety medication, and nausea medication should be taken as described on the bottles. The anxiety medicine can be useful to help you rest, relax, and whisper as described above.

## Eyelid massage:

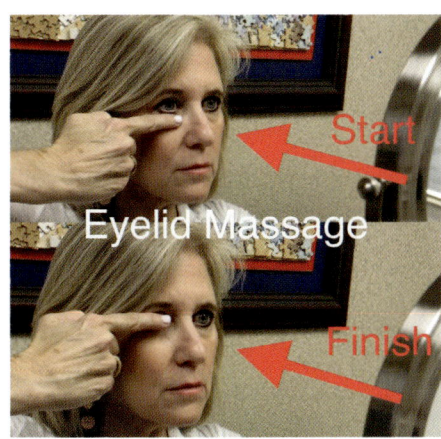

Eyelid Massage
Start
Finish

There's a video demonstrating eyelid massage on my webpage. This is ChrisSaundersMD.com, and this should be viewed at your convenience. Think of eyelid massage as a form of range of motion excise. If you had knee surgery, the doctor might send you to a physical therapist to maintain and to keep range of motion. There is no physical therapist for the eyes, except you and me. The upper eyes do not need massage because of the natural blink mechanism. The lower eyes are massaged to maintain this range of motion and to minimize any abnormal healing.

The eyelid massage is predominantly done in the *up direction*. The finger is used to elevate the lower eyelid going inwards slightly, but predominantly up. The force required should be on the moderate side. Don't be too hard with pressure causing bruising or injury. Too little pressure won't do anything. You will be instructed by me personally when to start this. The eyelid massage will also be shown to you in detail. Watch the video on my web page.

## Incisions:

Eye incisions are placed in one of the best areas of the body to heal. *These incisions most likely heal better than any place on the entire body!* They are privileged and almost uniformly heal extremely well and are difficult to see. This particular location is fantastic and is why we place the incisions in this location. The vast majority of patients need no scar creams or care for their incisions. Healing poorly is extremely unlikely.

## Exercise and Activity:

For the first week, most people should be at home. Walking around the house is the predominant activity allowed. As mentioned above, be careful about doing too much screen time as it can dry out the eyes and delay recovery. Usually after about 1 week, you're allowed to begin light activities and after 2 weeks unlimited activity. This is dependent upon your healing, and I will approve more activity during your recovery as you heal.

Chapter 17

# Rhinoplasty

## Summary

Rhinoplasty is the medical word for a nose job. The operation is performed to make the nose smaller, thinner, and more attractive in appearance. It is one of the most commonly performed cosmetic operations in America. It is also one of my favorite and one I specialize in. It is a very creative operation, and this is one of the reasons I like to do it. The lights of the operating room are dimmed low, and the only light is my headlight and magnifying glasses. It is an operation where you go slow and work meticulously.

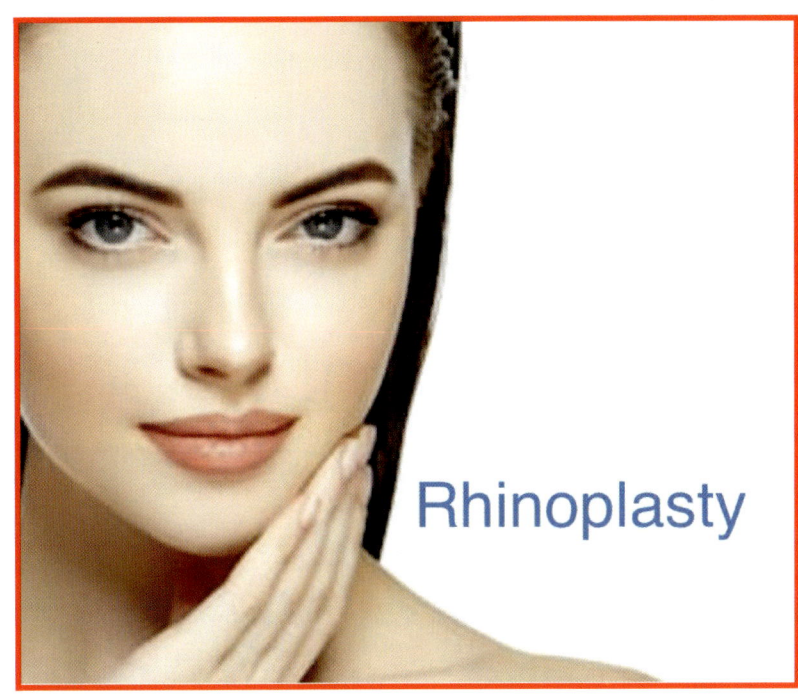

The recovery, like most facial operations, is characterized by very little pain but significant bruising and swelling. You must allow time to resolve the bruising. This is important to understand. It's like a hibernation period. The small amount of pain is reassuring to most. The internal packs are a nuisance but come out quickly. The splint stays on about a week. Satisfaction and results of this cosmetic operation tend to be very high. This chapter reviews the recovery from the operation rhinoplasty.

## Head Elevation:

It is important to keep the head elevated at all times. This includes sleeping. This can be done in a lounge chair or in bed. It should be at least 45° of head elevation; it is important to minimize bruising, swelling, and to aid healing.

## Rest, Relax, and Whisper:

This is a concept. Just like with other facial surgery operations such as facelifts and eye tucks, it's important to be calm and relaxed. Any type of increased activity or bearing down can lead to increased bleeding and delayed healing. Valsalva is the medical word for when humans bear down. Valsalvas are done with coughing, lifting heavy objects, talking loudly, screaming, yelling, and even laughing. All these activities should be avoided after a rhinoplasty. It's important to stay relaxed and calm to allow for bruising and swelling to go away as quickly as possible. Over doing it is a bad idea and can cause increased risks.

## Packs and Splints:

Antibiotic packs are placed inside the nose, and a splint is placed outside the nose. The nasal splint stays on for approximately 1 week. It is typically glued on at surgery and will remain secure for this timeframe. Some people with oily skin or who over do it might sweat off the splint. There's not much we can do to change the oil content of someone's skin. So don't over do it and sweat it off. Leave the splint alone, so we can get the best healing. Showers should not be too hot, as the steam will loosen up the splint too early.

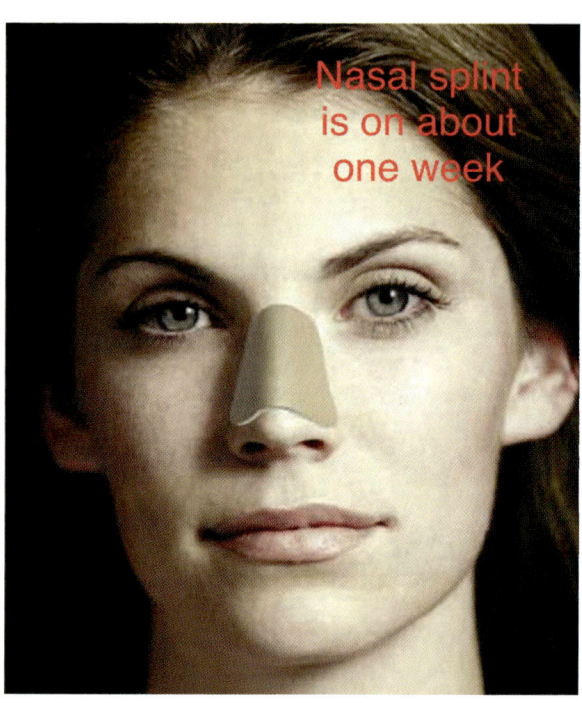

Nasal splint is on about one week

Antibiotic packs are placed at the time of surgery to minimize bleeding; they stay in approximately 24 to 48 hours, unless a septoplasty was performed at the same time. In this case, the packs stay in for an extra day or two. *Do not remove the pack.* This would be a big mistake! If the packs were to come slightly out, use a clean hand and finger to push it back in. It's easy and doesn't hurt. The packs are uncomfortable, but they do not cause pain. You do have to breathe through your mouth, and so it's not uncommon to have a dry or sore throat for a couple days after a rhinoplasty.

The packs are removed in the office by me or the nursing staff. There is minimal pain upon removal of the packs. So please don't worry. Most people will say it was, "no big deal."

## Bleeding and Bandages:

It's common to have some bloody drainage after a nose job. This can be out of the nose but also down the throat. Gauze is typically worn beneath the nose and is called a *drip pad*. The drip pad is changed as much as is necessary depending on the drainage. It might have to be changed 5 or 6 times the first day or evening following surgery. The next day will typically be much less and eventually the drainage goes down to zero. Some patients will also have bleeding in the back of their throat. Try not to swallow this blood. It's best to spit it out, so as not to upset your stomach.

Remember, the packs inside your nose are not to be pulled out by you. If they come out a bit, push them up with a clean finger. Removal is a very bad idea. *The drip pads beneath your nose can be changed as necessary*. More frequent changing is common the first day or two. The drainage and bleeding slowly stop over a couple of days. When you change the drip pad, sometimes it will stick and pull on the internal nasal pack. Remove the drip pad slowly and separate it from the internal packing, if necessary. This is easy and will stop accidental removal of the packs.

**Icing:**

Gentle icing of the surrounding area of the nose is permitted. Please do not try to ice the nose itself, as there are delicate stitches that could be disrupted. Ice can be applied 20 minutes on and 20 minutes off for the first 72 hours to the forehead and surrounding cheek areas.

**Showering:**

It's ok to shower the next day after surgery. As described above under splints, please do not take too hot a shower, as the steam will lead to the splint falling off. This could adversely affect your outcome. Showers should be cooler than normal and should be kept to a minimum. Do not have the water splash directly in your face.

**Medications:**

Take your antibiotics as prescribed. The antibiotics are mandatory and should be taken when you get home. If your stomach is upset, they can be started in the morning. The pain medication, anxiety medication, and nausea medication should be taken as prescribed on the bottle.

**Return to Work:**

It's normal to have bruising and swelling around the nose after a rhinoplasty. This can take several weeks to gradually go away. The splint typically comes off a week after surgery, and people can return to work shortly after that. Make-up can be worn to cover any bruising, as some people will notice your bruising upon return to work. If you are trying to be more confidential and hide the bruising, then you should probably wait 2 weeks before returning to work.

**Exercise and Activity:**

The first several days after surgery you should have extremely light activity, such as just walking around the house. Too much activity can stir up bleeding. Excessive activity can start bleeding from the internal nasal incisions. After 10 days, walking and additional light activity are allowed. After 3 weeks, unlimited activity is now permitted.

Chapter 18

# Liposuction and Brazilian Butt Lift

## Summary

Liposuction or liposculpturing is the process of removing excess and unwanted fat from the body. Common areas of liposuction are the stomach, love handles, and outer thighs. Brazilian Butt Lift (BBL) is the name given to an operation where fat is removed via liposuction from one location and transferred to the buttock. The purpose is to make the buttock area fuller, rounder, and more attractive. In contrast to many operations, liposuction and BBL have tiny little incisions that allow for the introduction of suction cannulas. The cannulas suck out the fat and allow transfer to the buttock. The operations are not scarless, but the incisions are extremely small. Most people are extremely happy with their new thinner, flatter, and attractive body. If a BBL is done, most love their fuller buttock.

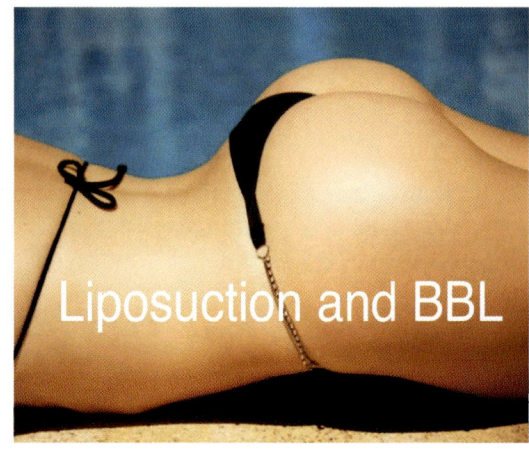

Liposuction is wonderfully easy. *The recovery surprises most people, in my opinion.* The pain is low and goes away very quickly. The next day after surgery, the vast majority of patients just feel sore. Many people are off pain medication in less than 24 hours. Full activity can be resumed in just 10 days.

BBL recovery involves not sitting on the buttock area to allow for the best healing and results. The recovery is not particularly more painful, just more difficult in that you must not sit on the buttock for about a month. Sitting causes pressure to the area and decreases blood supply. The sitting decreases *the take* or the amount of fat that survives. This is one of the main factors that determine results and patient satisfaction.

Loose skin must be considered. If you have loose skin in the stomach, then tummy tucks are probably a better choice. Older individuals and people who have had babies need to consider other operations and to understand that liposuction might not deliver the best results. The operation is discussed with you in detail during your consultation. This chapter will review the recovery from liposuction and/or BBL.

## Bandages:

The most modern types of liposuction involve the tumescent technique. This means that medicated fluid is injected into the areas, before the liposuction is performed. The injected medication typically has epinephrine and lidocaine. These help with decreasing bleeding and also with pain control. The tumescent fluid will, however, leak out to a degree after surgery, and the bandage will frequently become wet.

Just like one drop of blood in the toilet bowl, the fluid that leaks out is typically pink colored. Some patients can become alarmed by the drainage, but it is actually an extremely small amount of blood turning the fluid pink or reddish in color. This happens almost with all patients and is to be expected. If it becomes too wet, then the area that is wet can be reinforced with gauze. Clean hands should be used and do not touch any incisions. It is common for the bandages to be *wet*. As I have said, it is normal and to be expected because of the tumescent technique. It will dry over 24-36 hours.

Typically the patient is allowed to shower 48 hours after surgery. At the time of the shower, you should be in a bathrobe as the garment is washed and dried. The bandages do not need to be replaced after the shower.

**Bleeding or Drainage:**

As mentioned above, it might seem like a lot, but the actual blood loss from liposuction is extremely small. It tends to be pink or red colored, but the actual blood content is very little. Most of the bleeding or drainage stops in the first day or two. The drainage can stain car seats or chairs at home. Please be careful about what you sit on the first day or two. It's often common to use towels or old blankets beneath you to collect any drainage that you have after the procedure.

**Bruising:**

Bruising is at its peak 1-3 days after surgery. It gradually resolves over 2 weeks to a couple of months.

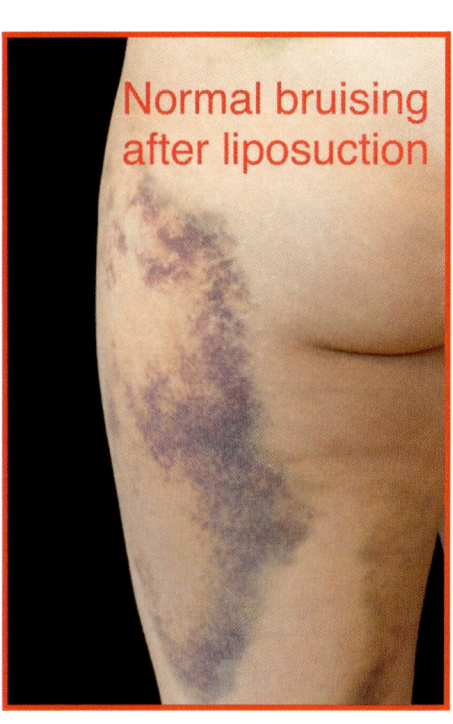

**Pain:**

Most people are surprised at how little pain they have after liposuction. *In my experience, it's very common for patients to say the next day after surgery that they are just sore.* Occasionally some people have more pain than I have just described. But it's important to understand that the vast majority of people will find that there is little to minimal pain after liposuction. This is great news for most. Pain prescription medication is provided for people with more severe pain. Most people can use just Tylenol or Motrin for their discomfort.

**Garments:**

You will be provided with a compression garment or binder that is placed on you after surgery. They should be worn as much as possible for approximately 6 weeks. You can be out of the garment for a short period of time to wash and dry it. If the surgery is performed in the hot summer months, it can be taken off for comfort and reapplied when you are in a cooler or air-conditioned location.

You are provided with a garment, but some people will choose to buy or obtain a second garment. This allows you to wear one while the second one is being washed. The fit of the garment is important. The concept is pressure where you had surgery. The garment can be any color or fabric, it just needs to be moderately tight. The pressure should not be too loose, and it should not be too tight, but a more medium tightness.

Many garments are crotchless to allow for easy urination without having to take the garments off. But this is an option, and it is not a required aspect of the garment. Spanx and Flexees are common brands of compression garments that I like.

**BBL:**

With a Brazilian Butt Lift, the fat is classically harvested from the stomach and the love handle areas. It is processed and transferred to your buttock. *The recovery involves predominantly keeping off the buttock area.* The pressure of

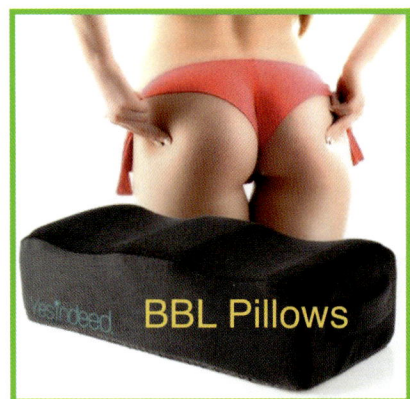

BBL Pillows

sitting decreases blood supply and the amount of fat that survives. Ultimately, this is one of the biggest factors that leads to the best results. Most doctors say keep off your buttock for 2 weeks. I believe the best results come from keeping off the buttock for 1 month.

There are *booty* pillows and buttock supports that can be purchased online. They are used to allow for some sitting that still keeps pressure off the buttock. Donut shaped pillows can help with this also. I will review these with you in detail to help you with this aspect of the recovery.

With liposuction, you can lie on the areas treated. After a BBL, you can lie on your sides or stomach. This is good and helps both the liposuction and the BBL areas heal.

**Blood Clot or DVT Prevention:**

As with all operations, early ambulation is an important instruction after liposuction. Early ambulation means getting up and walking around for approximately 10 minutes about 10 times a day. If there was thigh liposuction done, make sure the garment or girdle is not tight, constrictive, or bunched up in any particular area. This can happen around the knee area or in the thigh area. This type of bunched up garment can lead to an increased risk of blood clots. *Please read Chapter 5 on blood clot prevention to get more information on this extremely important topic.*

**Medications:**

The antibiotics are mandatory to take. You receive intravenous antibiotics before surgery to minimize risks of infection. Start your oral antibiotics when you get home. If your stomach is upset, you can start them the next day. The pain medicine, anxiety medicine, and nausea medicine should be taken as prescribed on the bottle.

**Return to Work:**

Most people can return to work in just a couple of days. Some people can return to work the day after liposuction. A long weekend is a classic recovery time for most patients. After this period you can resume light activities, driving, and work. After 10 days, patients can resume all activities and jobs, including strenuous exercise.

**Exercise and Activities:**

Light activity is recommended for the first 10 days. After 10 days, unlimited activity is allowed. The garment should be worn at all times, but for people having discomfort during exercise, they can remove the garment and reapply it after their exercise.

Chapter 19

# Body, Thigh, Arm, and Buttock Lifts

## Summary

Body, thigh, arm, and buttock lifts are done predominately to remove excess and unwanted skin and tissue from the respective areas. The operations are usually done for people with severe excess tissue that has come from weight loss, aging, or other causes of skin laxity. The benefits can be amazing and can provide high amounts of satisfaction for the proper individual. Results can transform a person with spectacular changes.

*However, it is important to understand the incisions, their location, and the length of the incisions.* This is an essential part of knowing these surgeries. These operations require long incisions. It is just a fact. Excess and loose skin of this magnitude will have to be cut out. This is the main and only way to remove it. Also, it's important to know that there are not any other options. There are no lasers, radio-frequency machines, or other techniques that will make a significant difference besides cutting out the loose skin. Other methods will just cost you money, and then you will be doing the lift anyway.

Because the main reason for these operations is just loose skin, the pain from the operations is not that bad. Since muscles don't have to be repaired, the pain is very manageable, and most people are surprised at the recovery process. Drains are a necessary part of these operations. Blood clots and their prevention must be understood in detail, and all preventative measures emphasized and strictly followed. This chapter describes recovery from these body lift procedures.

## Bandages:

The incisions are covered with bandages, and the patient is then typically placed into a body or compression garment. It is normal to have some bloody drainage. This is common, and it is frequently seen. It should be expected to a degree for most patients. The bandages are placed sterilely at the time of surgery and occasionally have to be reinforced. This should be done only for more than just a small amount of bleeding. If this is done, please do not touch the incisions, as this would potentially increase the risk of infection. If the bandages are reinforced, use clean hands and/or gloves, and do not touch the incision or where the drainage tubes come out the skin.

## Drains:

It's normal to have drainage tubes after these operations. They typically stay in approximately 1 week. The nurses will teach you how to take care of them, and they should be emptied approximately twice a day. Sometimes during the first couple of days, the drains will have to be emptied more frequently than twice a day. They might require emptying approximately 3 to 5 times a day. The output gradually diminishes over days. In general, I recommend the drainage tubes being emptied between 8 and 9 o'clock in the morning and then a second time between 8 and 9 o'clock at night. Record outputs of the drains on a piece of paper that can be shown to me during office visits. It is important to remember to squeeze the bulb flat after emptying the fluid. *It must be squeezed, because this gives the suction that allows for the fluid to be collected.*

Finally, it is common to have drainage around the tube. Drainage around the tube can be messy; but it is extremely common, and it is not to be of concern. Sometimes you will see small little blood clots in the tube themselves. These little clots can be *milked* along to help with drainage. Please don't touch where the drains come out the skin. Please be gentle doing this milking, so as to not injure or rip the tubes.

*Please read Chapter 14 on tummy tuck drains and their management. The drains are managed the same way for these lift operations.*

### Incisions:

The Steri-Strips are left on for approximately 1 week after surgery. After removal of the Steri-Strips, use Neosporin twice a day for 3 days, then use Bio-Oil twice a day. I have had excellent success with this product in helping the scars fade. Some patients will like to use silicone strips and silicon creams. I used these products for over 20 years and was not very impressed. I believe they are expensive and overrated. If somebody has them or chooses to use them, I do not object. If they had success with them in the past, it is also acceptable to use this product again. If you know they work for you, use them. I will keep a close eye on the fading of the incisions with you. Scars take approximately a year to fade. It is important to remember that time is required for complete fading of the incision.

### Blood Clots and DVT Prevention:

Early ambulation is an important instruction for all operations to minimize blood clot risks in the legs. Early ambulation means getting up and walking around the house for approximately 10 minutes about 10 times a day. Please make sure the garment is not too tight or bunched up in a given location. If it's bunched up, it could constrict blood supply in this area or cause a clot, and this would be unhealthy. Another method to minimize blood clot formation is patient positioning with the legs elevated above the heart. This is what I call *the tilted-back lounge chair.* By keeping the legs extremely elevated, it allows for better drainage and decreased clot formation. I also recommend *the invisible bicycle* to minimize blood clots. The legs are pumped frequently like riding a bicycle. This is done one leg at a time and can be done extremely frequently.

*It is mandatory to read Chapter 5 on blood clot prevention.* This will review in detail blood clots and their prevention.

### Showering:

You can shower after 72 hours or 3 days. No bathing or soaking is allowed. Only showers are permitted. At the time of the shower, all bandages are discarded, and the garment is typically washed and dried at this time. You can wear a bathrobe when the garment is being washed. Steri-Strips should not be removed at this time. They cover and protect the incision. Sometimes they lift up a bit. Try and leave them alone and not to disrupt them. They are left on until approximately 1 week and are described 2 paragraphs above on incisions. During your shower, please do not disrupt any drainage tubes and be careful with them.

It is common to feel lightheaded at the first shower, and it is recommended to have someone help you with the shower. You should also have a sitting stool. If you feel lightheaded, please sit down and rest. It will usually pass in 5 to 10 minutes, and you'll feel normal again. After the shower, no gauze is necessary for the incision has sealed. After the garment has been washed, it should be placed back on. Please make sure it's not bunching up at a given location. It is not necessary to reapply gauze as stated; but some people will feel comfortable doing so.

A T-shirt or other cotton shirt can be worn to apply padding to the lower abdominal incisions. This is comfortable and recommended. The drains should be refastened to the garment to avoid them being accidentally pulled out.

## Activity:

Please see blood clot prevention Chapter 5 mentioned above. Initially, activity is described as *up and about* which means early ambulation and walking around the house to minimize blood clot formation. As we heal, activity can be increased. No twisting or turning from side to side at the waist. This twisting can cause the abdominal skin to move over the deeper layers and lead to increased fluid production. This is important for the first month and after that period normal twisting can be done.

As we heal, activity can be increased based upon follow up visits with me in the office. Typically for the first week to two, light activity is recommended which means predominantly walking around the house as described. Between 2 and 6 weeks, I describe it as a *phased-in* recovery. This means activity can be increased as described. From 2 to 6 weeks usually stationary bicycles, ellipticals (no arm moving), and walking on a treadmill are acceptable activities. Strenuous activity is not done for 6 weeks. After 6 weeks, unlimited activity is allowed.

*Arm lifts or brachioplasty surgery has special activity instructions.* The arms should be kept as straight as possible for the first week. If you bend the arms at right angles, it could decrease blood supply and hinder healing, as the bandage can bunch up at the elbows. Reading tends to be an arm position with bent arms, so be careful when reading after surgery. Also, as with all operations, be gentle and careful when moving. Arm movement above the head (to reach a cabinet for example) could disrupt the arm incisions. Be wise and limit movement of the arms, in particular overhead.

## Medications:

The antibiotics are mandatory, and you start these when you get home. Intravenous antibiotics are given before surgery to decrease infection risks. If your stomach is upset, you can start the oral antibiotics in the morning. The pain medication, nausea medicine, and anxiety medicine should be taken as described on the bottle. Tylenol and Motrin are acceptable additional medications that can be taken for pain.

## Return to Work:

Most patients can return to work approximately 10 to 14 days after surgery. It is, however, possible to do work at home on the computer or with the laptop almost as soon as you feel able to do so. You must follow blood clot prevention methods as described. *You can not sit at a desk, as this would lead to an increased risk of blood clots.* If you are doing work on a computer or laptop, you should still be in the position described above to minimize risks of blood clots. This would mean that the laptop would probably be on your stomach with your legs elevated, during any work being performed at home.

Some patients will like to use silicone strips and silicon creams. I used these products for over 20 years and was not very impressed. I believe they are expensive and overrated. If somebody has them or chooses to use them, I do not object. If they had success with them in the past, it is also acceptable to use this product if they know it works for them. I will keep a close eye on the fading of the incisions with you. Scars take approximately a year to fade. It is important to remember that time is required for complete fading of the incision.

Chapter 20

# Breast Lift and Breast Reduction

## Summary

The medical word for breast lift is mastopexy. The medical words for a breast reduction are a reduction mammoplasty. *These operations are designed to elevate, lift, and enhance the appearance and the shape of the breasts.* In both operations, the nipples are elevated and the breast is reshaped to give it a more attractive and natural appearance. Reductions also have the purpose of making the breasts significantly smaller in volume or size. This is one of the main goals of reductions. With breast lifts, the volume can be decreased by any amount desired by the woman. The lift can be just very small decreases in size or larger amounts if wanted. Breast lift/reduction recovery is distinctly different from breast augmentation recovery. The best news about breast lifts and reductions is there is substantially less pain involved than using breast implants.

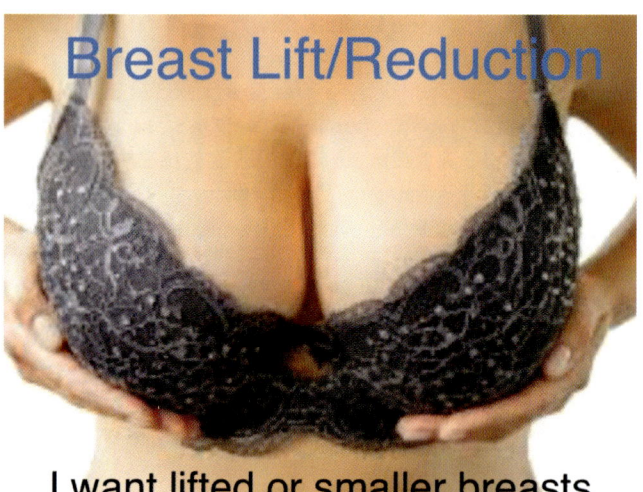

The reason there is substantially less pain is because the surgery involves no muscle work. The vast amount of surgical pain from operations comes from bones, ribs, cartilage, and muscles. Surgery on human *flesh* is characterized by substantially less pain. The breast is obviously extremely important and is one of the most sexual and sensual parts of our body. But the good news is, it actually does not have as much pain as most people would expect, and recovery is easy for many because no muscle work is done.

Breast lifts are done to elevate and reshape the breasts. The woman has the choice of being slightly smaller, or she can choose a larger decrease in size. This is her choice, and it is reviewed by me in detail in your consultation. Some women might want to add implants. This can lead to an elevated breast and give extra fullness that the lift alone will not do. Breast reductions essentially are lifts where large amounts of tissue are removed. This can be covered by insurance companies for pain related to large breasts. It can be difficult to get insurance coverage, however, and they will require extremely large amounts of breast tissue removed.

This chapter focuses on these wonderful operations with the goals of elevating the breasts to give a higher, perkier, and more attractive shape.

## Bandages:

Patients will have Steri-Strips on the incisions covered with gauze pads, and an Ace-wrap bandage is wrapped around the breasts and chest. It's normal for the bandage to feel snug. Please do not loosen or tighten this bandage, as it has been personally wrapped by me. If for some reason the bandage slips down or becomes disrupted, it can be gently rewrapped. It is safer to be on the loose side than the tighter side. If this is required, do not touch the incisions, as this could increase your risk of complications. Some doctors use surgical bras instead of the Ace-wrap. I have found these to be *one size fits no one*. I have found the Ace-wraps to be easy and vastly superior for comfort and recovery.

It is normal to have some drainage and spotting of blood on the bandages. This is most common on the sides. This is a typical occurrence after surgery. Do not worry. Almost everyone has this happen afterwards.

## Bleeding:

As mentioned above, it is normal to have some spotting of blood on the sides of the bandages. Please do not be alarmed. Occasionally, this can be more than a small amount. One side will almost always have more blood than the other side. It is ok to reinforce the bandage if necessary. This usually means applying extra gauze on top of the old gauze, instead of replacing it. If you do this, please have freshly washed hands and/or wear gloves. Please don't touch the incisions, as this can increase chances of infection. The next morning bandages will be changed during your postoperative visit to the office.

## Showering:

You should keep the incisions dry for 72 hours or 3 days. After 3 days you can take your first shower. At this time remove all gauze, and the Ace bandage is discarded. Do not disrupt the Steri-Strips. The Steri-Strips can be gently removed after approximately 1 week. An old-fashioned instruction is to leave the Steri-Strips on until they fall off. I do not recommend this. After removal of the Steri-Strips, you should use Neosporin twice a day for 3 days and then start Bio-Oil twice a day. Showering is permitted and recommended daily after the first 3 days. No bathing or hot tubs are permitted for 6 weeks.

## Pain Pump and Pain Buster:

In contrast to breast augmentation, breast lifts and reductions do not have that much pain, so the pain pump or Pain Buster is not used. Some people will be disappointed by this. But, it's actually good news. There really is not that much pain. The pain is very manageable with medication only. Most people are surprised by how little pain there is. If you have a breast lift and a breast augmentation, you will receive a pain pump; because the breast implant causes more discomfort. Please see Chapter 10 to read about the recovery from breast augmentation and Chapter 7 to read about the Pain Buster.

## Medications:

The antibiotics are mandatory to take after surgery. You will receive intravenous antibiotics for prophylaxis before surgery to minimize the risks of infection. Start the oral antibiotics when you get home, or the next morning if your stomach is upset. The other prescribed medications are taken on an as necessary basis. The pain medication, anxiety medication, and nausea medicine are taken if you are experiencing these problems. Motrin and Tylenol are acceptable medications to be taken after surgery to help with any discomfort.

## Drains:

I do not use surgical drains after these operations. They are not necessary in my experience and opinion.

**Breast Massage:**

Breast massage is not needed for breast lifts and reductions. If you have a breast augmentation, in addition to your breast lift, then please review Chapter 11 on breast augmentation massage. There is no breast massage for patients having just a breast lift or a breast reduction.

**Return to Work:**

Many patients can return to work and light activities after 3 to 5 days. One week off is a classic recovery period. Most can resume light activities, work, and driving in this time frame. After these operations, if people have more time off from work then 2 to 4 weeks off is nice. But, it's not usually necessary for most patients.

**Bras:**

After your first shower at 3 days, you should wear a sports bra. I call it *an old fashioned sports bra with no underwires, no paddings, and no built in cups.* It should be moderately snug. This means that it should not be too tight or too loose. The sports bra is typically worn for approximately 1 month. After a month, you can purchase any bra desired including underwires. This can be done after approval by me during one of your follow up visits.

**Incisions:**

The incisions are initially covered by Steri-Strips. Steri stands for sterile, and they are placed at the end of the operation. As mentioned above, they should be removed by you after approximately 7 days. They do not need to be left on longer, as this is old-fashioned. After the strips are removed, please use Neosporin twice a day for 3 days. After this please start Bio-Oil twice a day to help the incisions fade.

I recommend Bio-Oil for all the incisions. I have had excellent success with Bio-Oil and recommended it strongly.

Some patients will like to use silicone strips or silicone scar cream. I have no objection to these products. I have actually used them in the past for probably 20 years and personally was unimpressed by the results. I think they are expensive and overrated. But if a patient has had success with them in the past, and we know that they work for them personally, then I would recommend they continue to use these products.

**Exercise and Activity:**

Walking, driving, and returning to work is usually allowed after 3 to 5 days. 1 week is a classic amount of time before beginning walking as a light activity outdoors. It is important to keep activity minimal or light for approximately 2 weeks. The time between 2 and 6 weeks after surgery is described by me as a *phased-in* recovery period. Activity allowed during this period would include things like stationary bicycles, ellipticals without using the arms, and walking on a treadmill. More aggressive exercise like running, weights, and CrossFit are not allowed. All activities are permitted after 6 weeks and are encouraged.

Chapter 21

# Botox and Dysport

## Summary

Botox is a wonderful treatment that helps with wrinkles around the eyes, eyebrows, and in the forehead. The medications are called neuromodulators. The procedure is done in the office with minimal bruising in the vast majority of patients. Most people can resume normal activities and work the day after the procedure.

Patients usually have no complications or problems after Botox treatments. Last year there were 17 million minor procedures in America, including Botox and Dysport. These statistics are from the American Society of Plastic Surgery. This huge number of treatments underscores its' high success and extremely low risk.

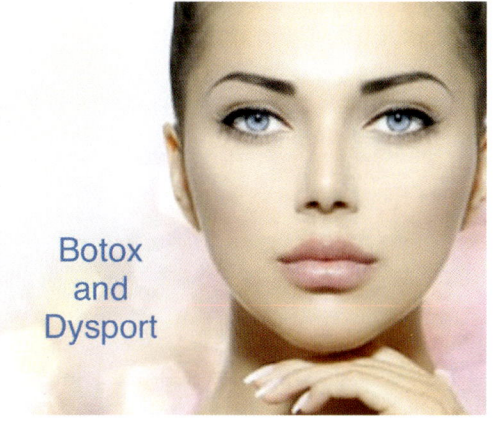

Botox
and
Dysport

It is still important to have realistic expectations about Botox treatments. Botox might not last as long as you hope, and it doesn't completely get rid of all wrinkles. Some patients might require a small *touch up* that would be done in the office to give the results an extra boost. Typically, there is no charge for this type of touch up. In general, as I have said, Botox improves wrinkles but does not "eliminate them" or "get rid of them."

Botox also might not last as long as desired. The product typically lasts around 3 months. Sometimes your body metabolizes the product more quickly and results diminish early. If this happens, you aren't harmed. The answer is to do more Botox. Some patients will choose to do smaller amounts of Botox than recommended, so as to save money. They should expect that the results will not last as long as if they had used larger quantities of Botox.

As I have already stated, results are usually excellent with high satisfaction. Risks are minimal and focus on minor bruising and swelling. *Patients must have realistic expectations and understand that the Botox only improves us.* It does not make us perfect, and Botox only lasts so long, approximately 3 months. It can be metabolized and go away more quickly.

## Bruising, Swelling, and Ice:

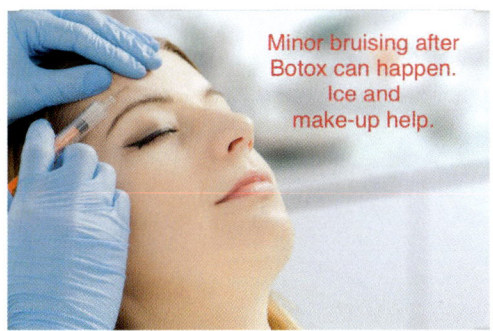

Minor bruising after Botox can happen. Ice and make-up help.

Recovering from Botox is extremely easy. Most people have minimal to no bruising and can resume normal activities the next day. Uncommonly, some people will get unlucky and get more significant bruising. Although disappointing, it is important to understand that it will not affect the results of the Botox. The Botox will still work normally. It will just take longer for the bruising to go away. Make-up can be used during this time to hide the bruising after the treatment.

It is recommended that icing be done to the treated areas for the first 3 days. I recommend that you ice 20 minutes on and 20 minutes off.

This should be done approximately 5 times a day. Additional icing can be done if needed and/or desired.

### Headache:

Headaches are one of the most common problems after Botox. They are usually minor and are located at the site of the injection. They usually go away quickly. I recommend Tylenol or Motrin for this headache pain.

### Redness, Welts, and itching:

Minor redness, welts, or itching can occur at treatment sites. This is common, minor, and of minimal significance, because they just go away. You should not worry. Benadryl cream or pills taken orally is recommended for these symptoms.

### Lumps and Swelling:

Patients will sometimes have minor lumps at the injection site. This is typically from minor bruising and/or swelling. Gentle icing as described above is recommended 20 minutes on and 20 minutes off for up to 3 days.

### Drooping of the Eyebrows or Eyelids:

Drooping of the eyebrows or eyelids is very uncommon, and most people do not get this problem. If you do, do not worry and please call the office for an appointment with me. The drooping will spontaneously resolve or go away on its own. Sometimes I will prescribe an eye drop medication which can help the condition resolve more quickly.

Some patients have droopy eyebrows to begin with before the procedure. Others might have extra skin in the eyelid area before the treatment. They might benefit from a blepharoplasty to improve this condition. In this case it's not a problem of the Botox but just overall aging of the eyelid, that would be better treated with cosmetic surgery. This would be discussed in detail with me on an office visit.

In general, drooping of the eyebrows and/or eyelids is rare. If it does occur, it will resolve gradually on its own.

### Results:

Please remember to have realistic expectations about Botox or Dysport. Like any cosmetic procedure, it is necessary to have a good understanding of what the treatment will do for you. *People can be disappointed if they expect the wrinkles to be completely gone versus just improved.* Botox is a chemical that works to diminish facial lines. It does take several days to reach its maximum potency or to *kick in*. This means that patients will typically see the best results approximately 3 to 5 days after treatment.

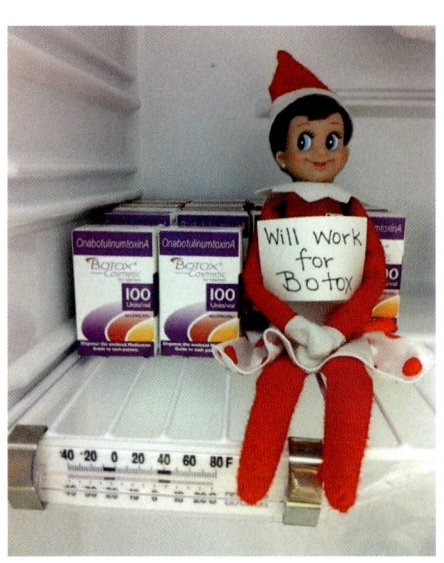

Botox lasts approximately 3 months. However, this can be from 6 weeks to 6 months for some. A lot of it is dependent on how quickly your body metabolizes the Botox. If the product does not last as long as it's desired, it's not the fault of the injector, but more related to how much Botox was used and how quickly your body metabolizes it. You aren't hurt or harmed if

this happens, just potentially disappointed that the Botox went away more quickly than desired. If this happens, the answer often is just to do a little more Botox to get more improvement or to use more Botox the next time you do a treatment.

I believe it is important that patients know how much Botox or how much Dysport was used in each area treated. If they know how many units of the product was used, they can help with future treatments. For example, if you receive 25 units of Botox in the forehead and don't get enough benefit, the next time more medicine should be used. Some people have larger muscles that need more medication. Some people metabolize a product faster and need more medicine. By understanding and remembering how much is used, you can help yourself with your treatments. Of course, we document how much is used and have this information available in case needed.

### How Long Does It Last?

I reviewed this topic in the paragraph above under results. However, it is an important topic, so I will repeat some key features. Botox lasts approximately 3 months. Some people will have results that only last 6 weeks and others will have Botox that lasts 6 months. This is often determined by how quickly your body metabolizes the product and how much Botox is injected. If the Botox goes away quicker than expected, it's not the injector making a mistake. It is the factors that I have described above.

If the Botox or Dysport goes way too quickly, the answer usually is to do an additional treatment or touch-up. This often leads to much higher satisfaction and success. I strongly recommend this.

### Return to Work:

Most patients can return to work immediately. There might be some minor visible bruising that can be diminished with ice application and/or make-up. If someone is worried about visible bruising, then typically they should go home and do frequent icing and return to work the following day.

### Activity:

It is allowed to return to full activities the day after the procedure. It is not recommended to exercise on the day of the procedure.

Chapter 22

# Facial fillers:   Restylane, Juvederm, and Sculptra

## Summary

Facial fillers are products used to improve wrinkles in the face, mainly around the mouth, lips, and eyes. They are also used for rejuvenation of the cheeks, jawline, and forehead. Fillers are great for lip enlargement. These products are some of the most commonly performed cosmetic procedures in the United States every year. Last year, coupled with other minimally invasive procedures, there were over 17 million performed! This was reported by the American Society of Plastic Surgery. They are *procedures* in contrast to surgical operations that might require being put to sleep. Facial fillers are typically done in the office on an outpatient basis.

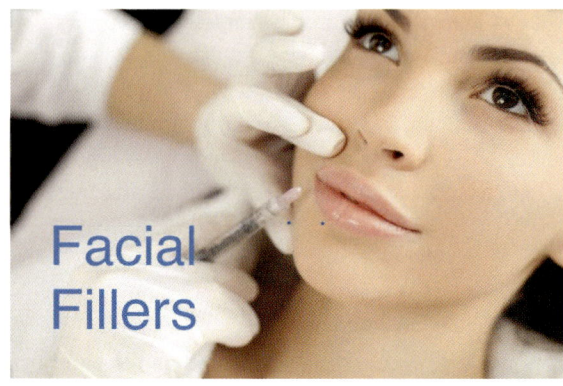

Fillers can be thought of as human spackle or putty. They are used *to fill* wrinkles, just as spackle would be used to fill up a crack in your wall. They are modern day collagen products that last much longer. Risks of the filler injections are extremely low. Statistically, they are one of the safest procedures you can do. However, the injections do cause bruising and swelling. This is part of the recovery. Most people get minimal bruising, but every once in a while someone gets more than the typical little bruising. This is not from error, but more just bad luck. The good news is that the bruising will still go away, and these people still get the benefits and results.

Satisfaction tends to be extremely high. This is why millions and millions do it. However, not everyone is happy. Dissatisfaction is uncommon but is usually from not getting as much benefit as hoped for. This means the wrinkle didn't *go away*. Or the product didn't last *as long* as desired. Realistic expectations are important. *These products improve us: they don't make us perfect.* They tend to diminish wrinkles, not "get rid of them." This is the most important thing to understand about fillers. Risks are extremely low, but they only help us. They don't make us a model or a movie star. This chapter will review the recovery from facial fillers.

## Bruising, Swelling and Ice:

Recovering from fillers such as Restylane, Juvederm, and Sculptra usually is very easy. Most people have minimal to

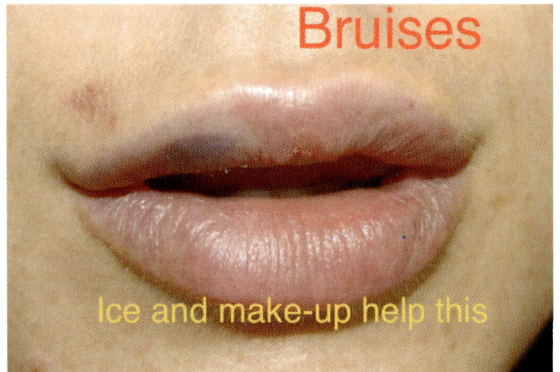

no bruising, and they can resume normal activities the next day. Occasionally, some people will get unlucky and have more swelling and bruising. Although disappointing, it is important to

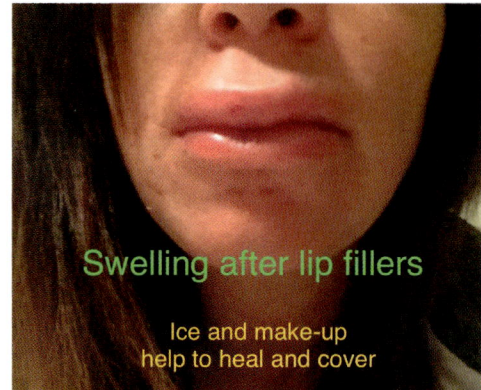

understand that it will not affect the results of the filler. It just will take longer for the bruising to resolve. Make-up can be used to hide the bruising following these procedures.

It is recommended that icing be done to the treated areas for the first 3 days. I recommend to ice 20 minutes on and 20 minutes off. This should be done approximately 5 times a day. Extra icing can be beneficial.

## Headache or Pain:

It is common to have minor headaches and/or pain at the injection site. This is common after fillers. The pain, however, is usually extremely little or very minor and goes away quickly. I have had these filters done many times to myself and although there is some pain during the injection process, I had essentially no pain afterwards. Some people will be more sensitive and have a little more pain then I have just described. Tylenol or Motrin is recommended for this minor pain and/or headache.

## Redness and Itching:

Minor redness and itching can occur at the injection site. This is very common, and you should not be concerned. Benadryl is recommended for this problem, and it can be taken orally or as a cream. I have had excellent success using this treatment.

## Lumps and Bumps:

This sounds scary, but it's actually minor and very common following injections of facial fillers. They resolve extremely quickly. Most lumps are just fluid or some minor bruising from the injection, and will go away quickly. If you feel lumpy spots, you can gently *massage* the spots. Push on the spot with continual pressure but gentle pressure for approximately 2 minutes. Repeat this 5 times a day. This is called massage and helps resolve bruising, swelling, or any lumpiness that might occur. Although extremely rare, people can get lumps or bumps that are more significant and don't go away. In my experience and in my office, this is very unlikely. In this unlikely event of a long lasting lump, it can be dissolved with a product called hyluronidase. This is easy and works very well for people who need the product dissolved. Basically, if you don't like your filler, it can just be dissolved with a minor injection. This is extremely helpful if needed.

## Results:

It is extremely important to have realistic expectations about the results of facial fillers. Most patients are very happy with these products when used for the cheeks, lips, and facial lines. *However, fillers do not get rid of all your wrinkles.* People should expect improvement but not complete wrinkle removal. If a patient doesn't get the results they desire, often the answer is to use more filler. This gives more benefit to the desired area. Some people also should be aware that surgery might be a better choice than facial fillers. Both are done for facial rejuvenation, but they are very different treatments.

If the results aren't as much as you want or desire, sometimes a cosmetic facelift or an eyelid tuck might be another choice or a better option. The surgery can give rejuvenation that facial fillers can not do. They can make you look much younger in a bigger way than fillers. This would be discussed by me in detail in a consultation in the office, reviewing your rejuvenation choices.

## How Long Do They Last?

Fillers are gradually absorbed and typically last approximately 1 year. A risk of the procedure is they don't last as long as it's desired. Some products last longer than a year, but for the majority of fillers, the visible benefit is going to be 6 to 12 months. Sculptra can last longer. The use of this longer-lasting filler should be discussed in person during a consultation. It does however require several treatments to work best.

How long fillers last is not dependent on the injector or the doctor. It depends on how quickly your body absorbs the product. If it's absorbed too quickly, it isn't someone doing something wrong; it's just a fact of how quickly your body metabolizes this product. In this case, it could be disappointing, but nothing is actually wrong. Additional product can be purchased and added to what you have done to get a better result and increased satisfaction.

## Return to Work:

Most patients can return to work the day after the procedure. There might be some visible bruising that can be diminished with ice and covered with make-up. Patients are allowed to return to work the next day.

## Activities:

You can return to full activities the day after the procedure. It is not recommended to exercise the day of the procedure. Icing is recommended to decrease bruising, and this should be done for 3 days. Make-up can be worn as necessary.

Chapter 23     BEFORE AND AFTER PHOTOS

## Breast Augmentation Case 1

Front, angle, and side views

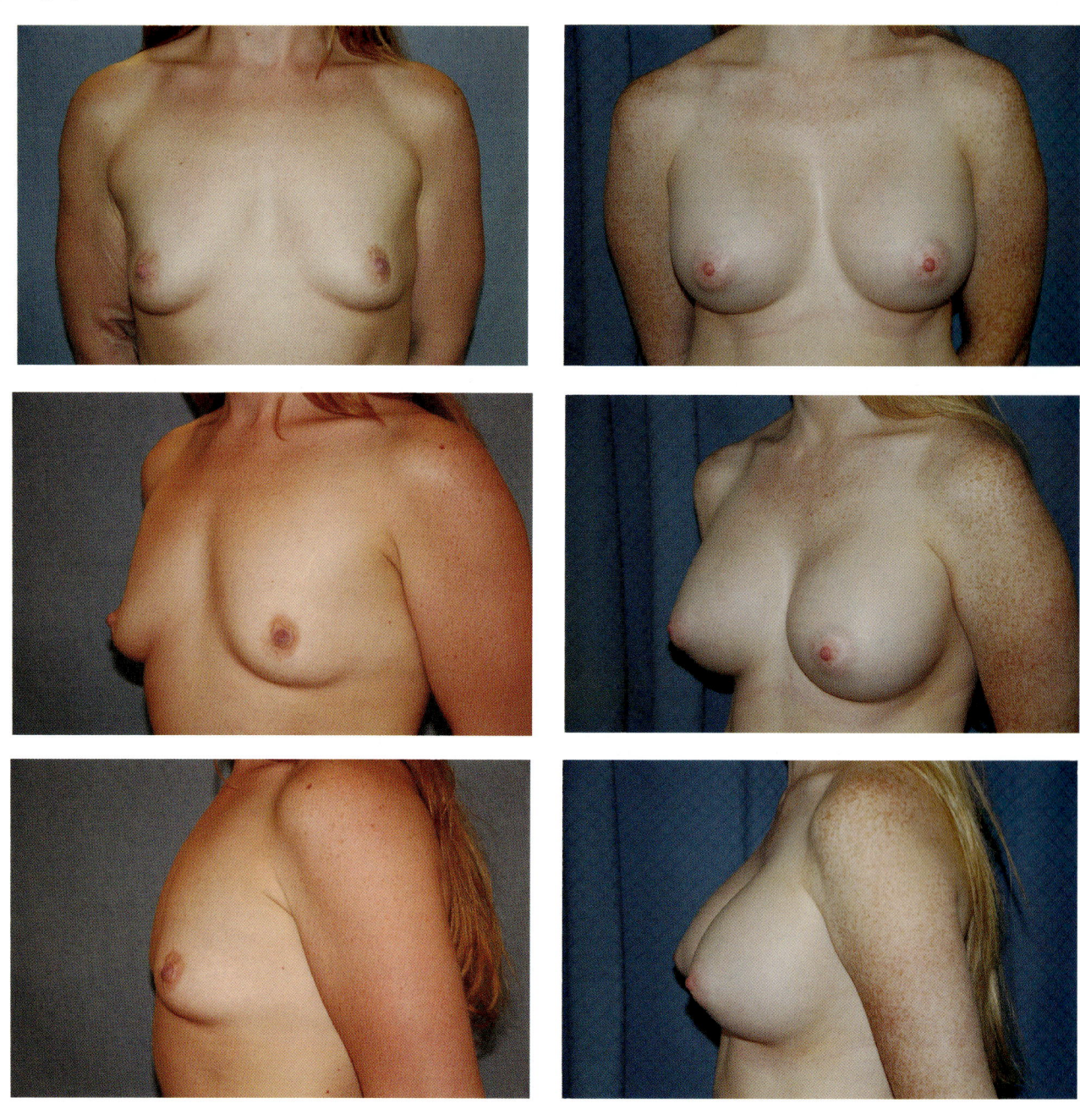

# Breast Augmentation Case 2

Front, angle, and side views

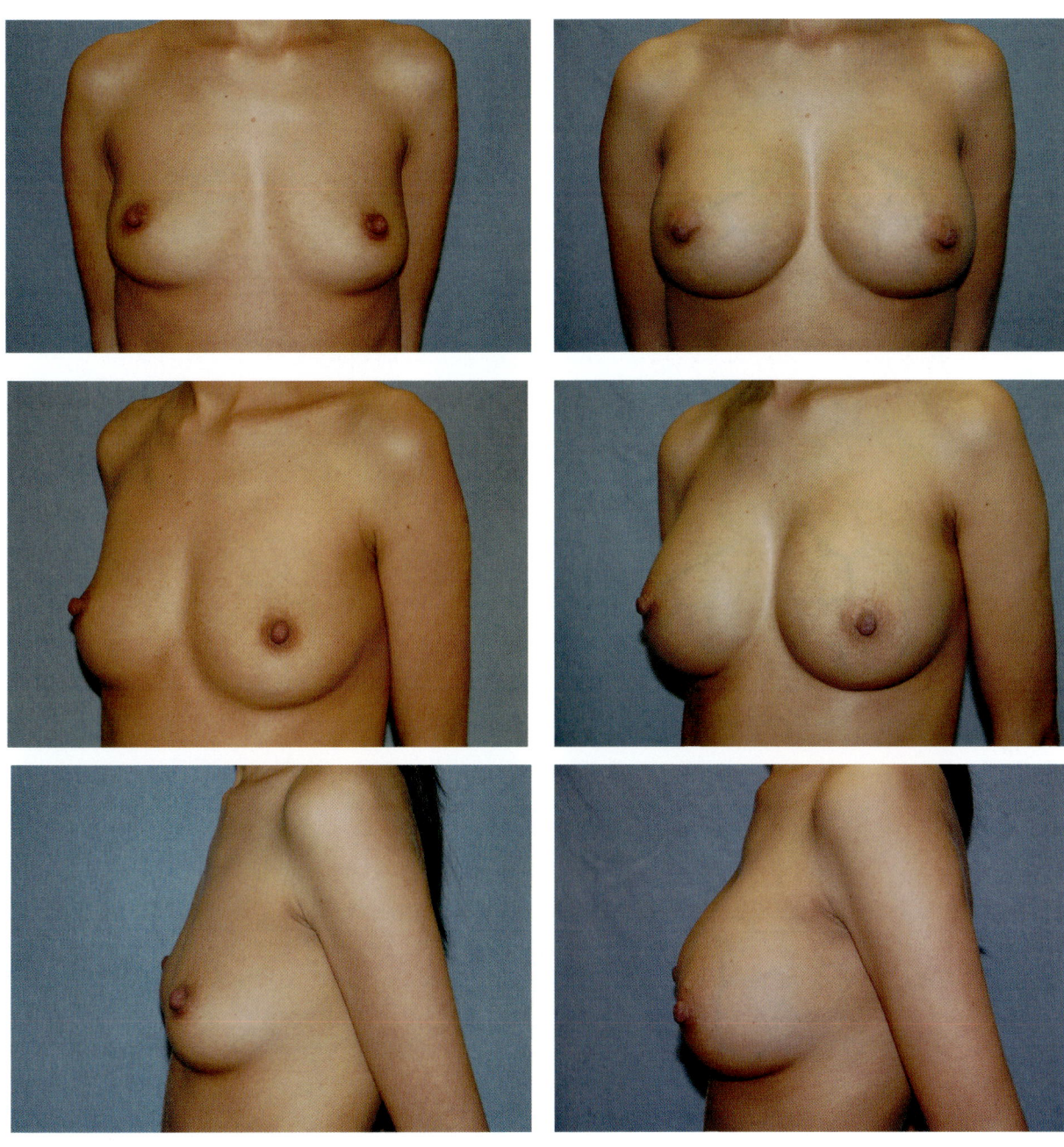

# Breast Augmentation Case 3

Front, angle, and side views

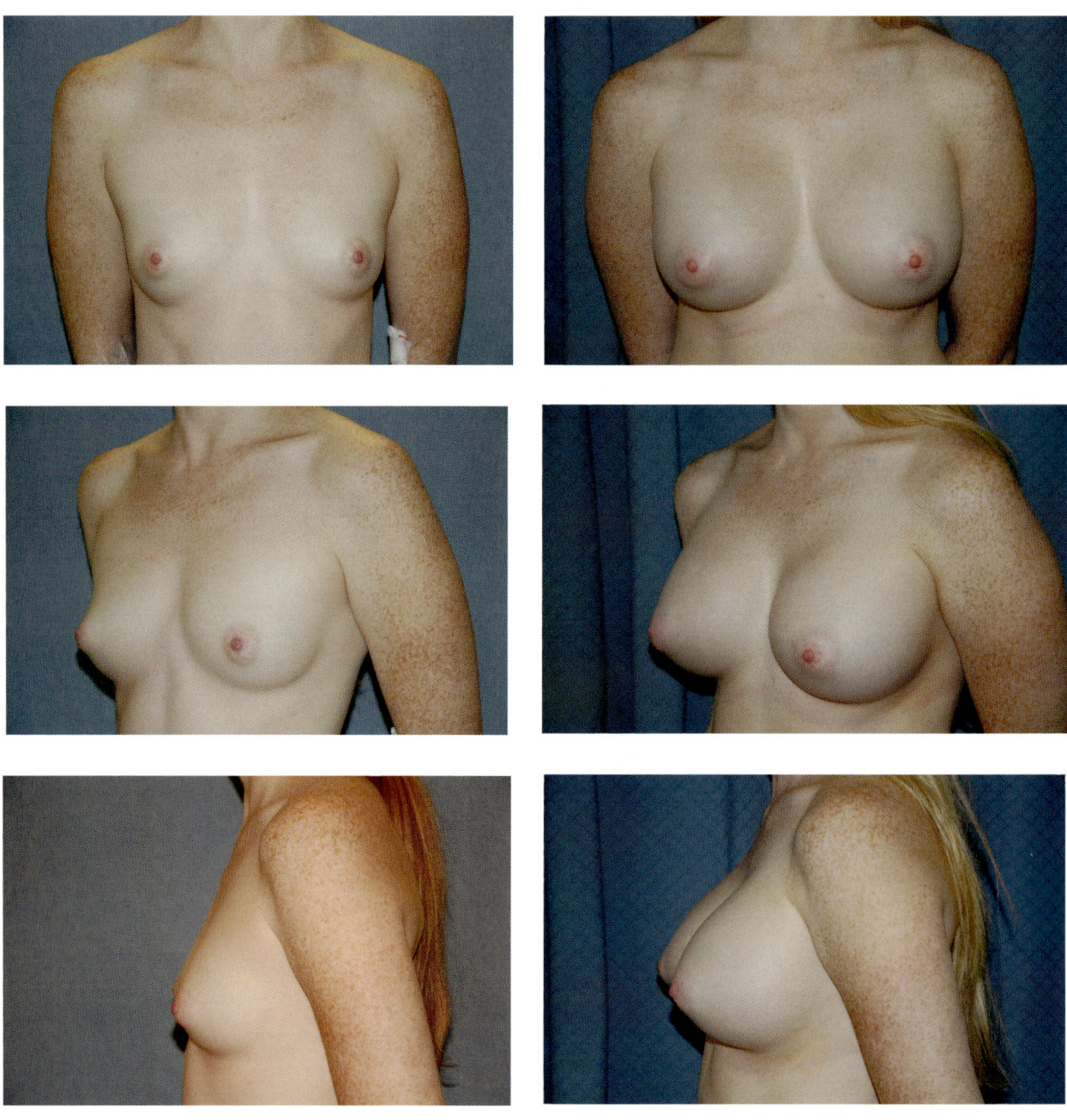

# Breast Augmentation and Breast Lift  Case 1

Front, angle, and side views

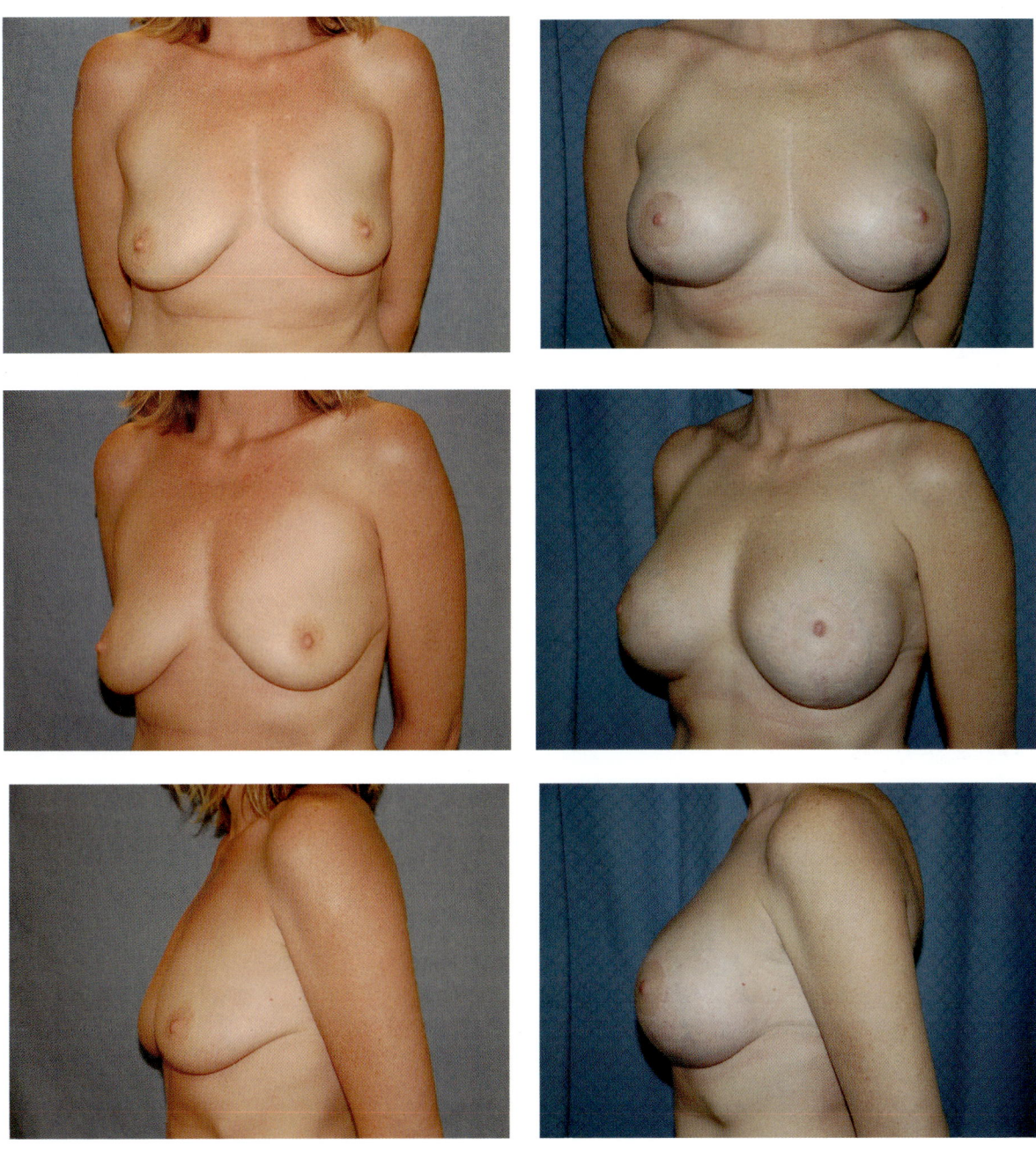

# Breast Augmentation and Breast Lift Case 2

Front, angle, and side views

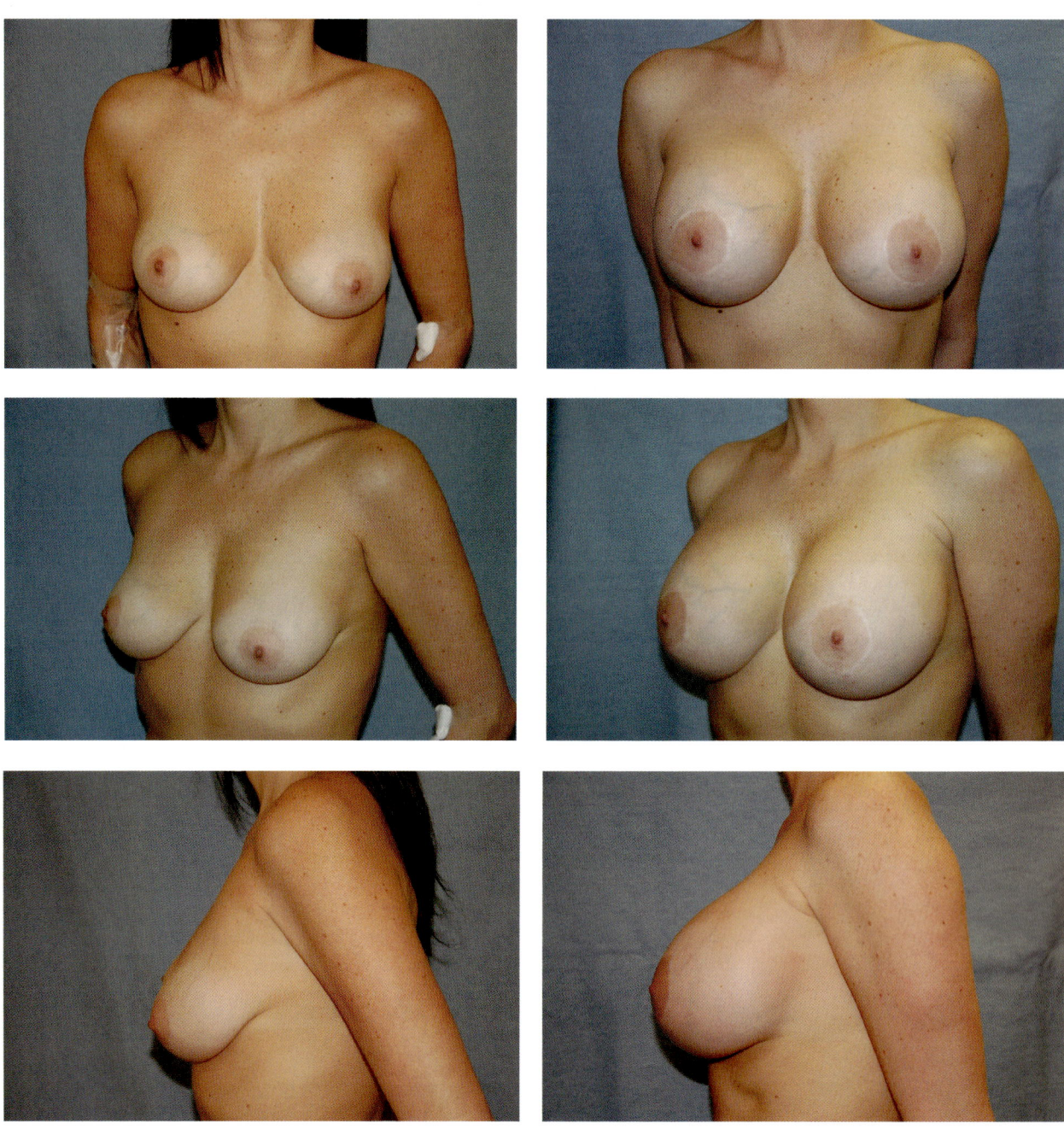

# Breast Augmentation and Breast Lift Case 3

Front, angle, and side views

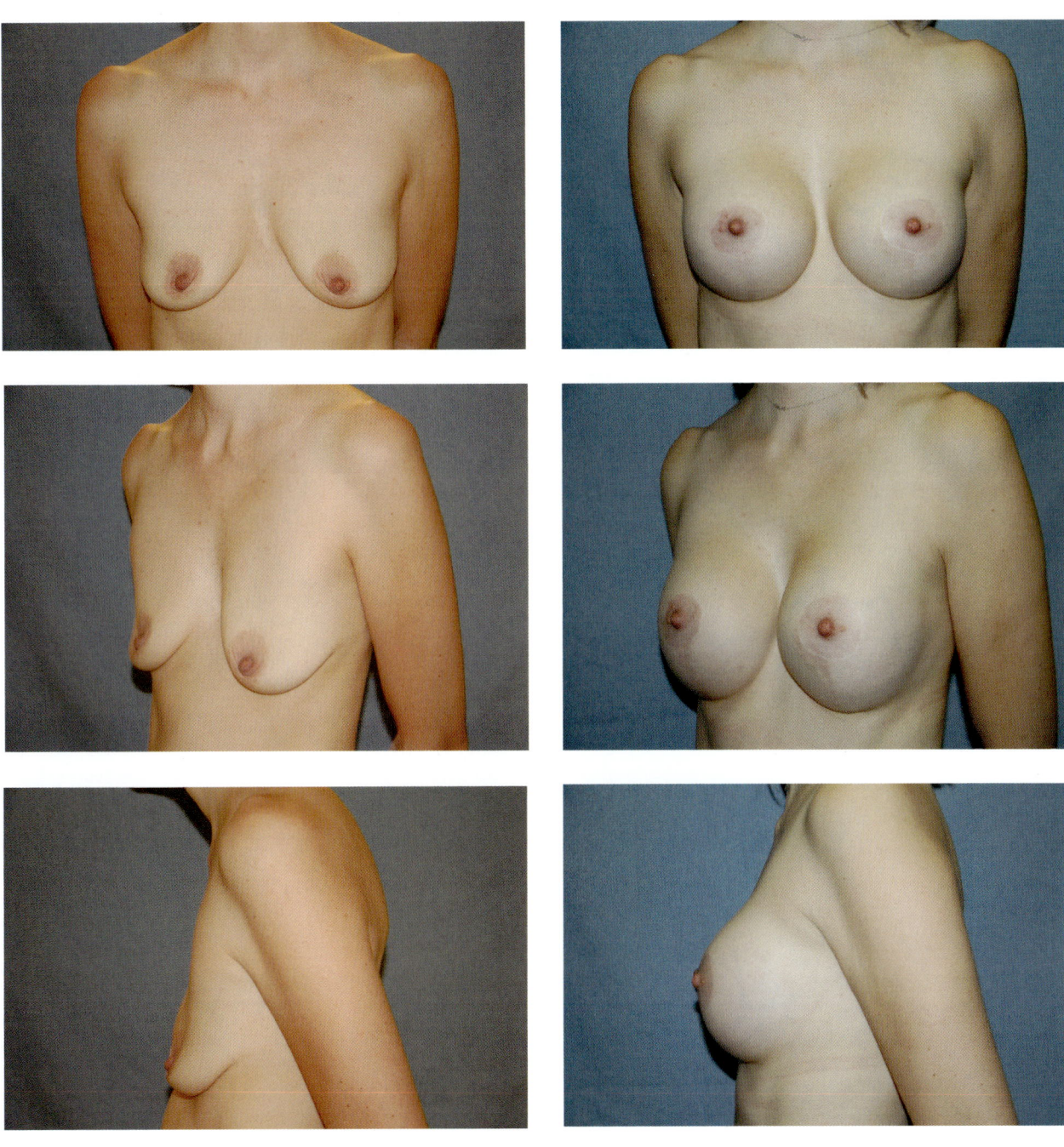

## Mommy Makeover Case 1

Angle view

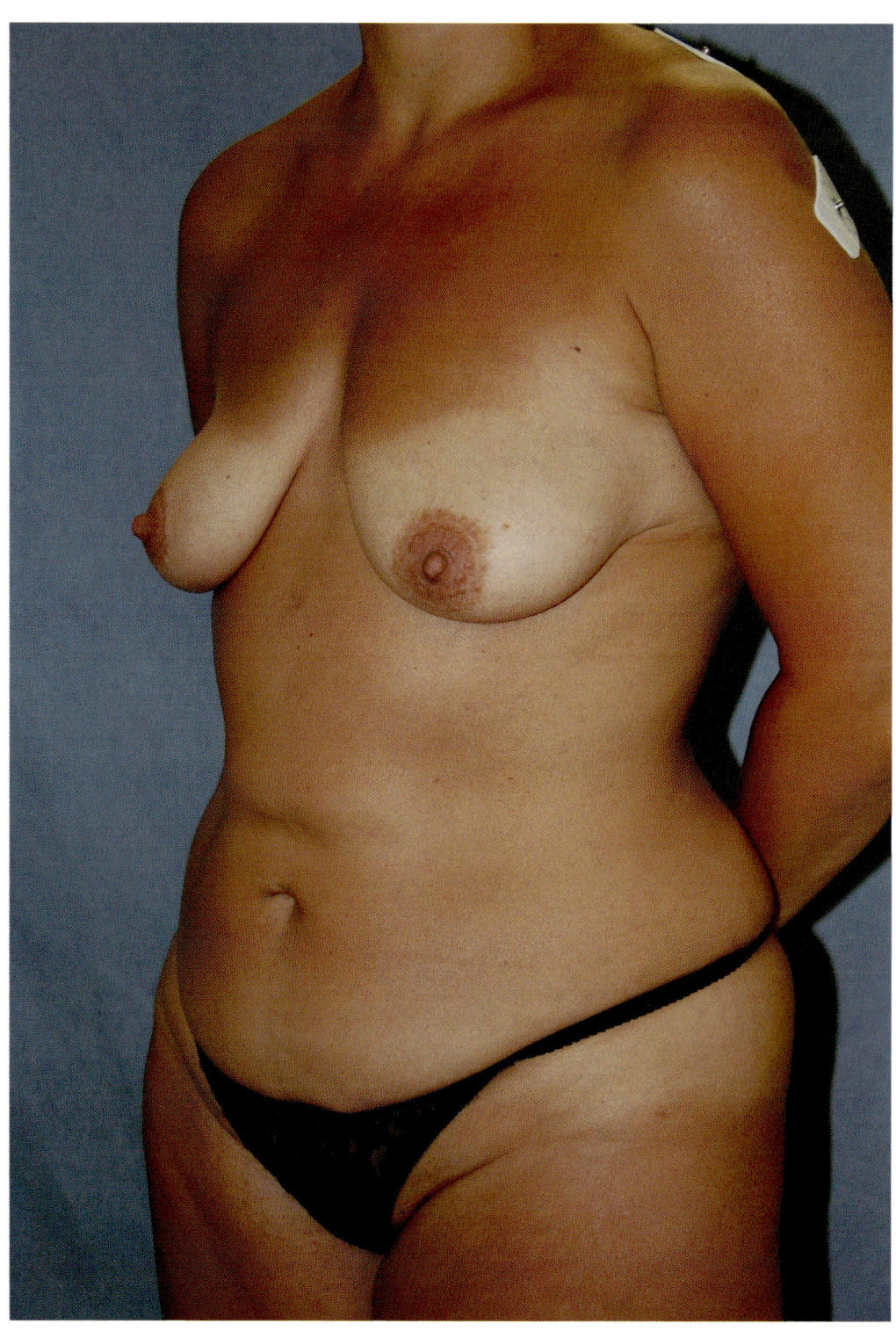

Angle view

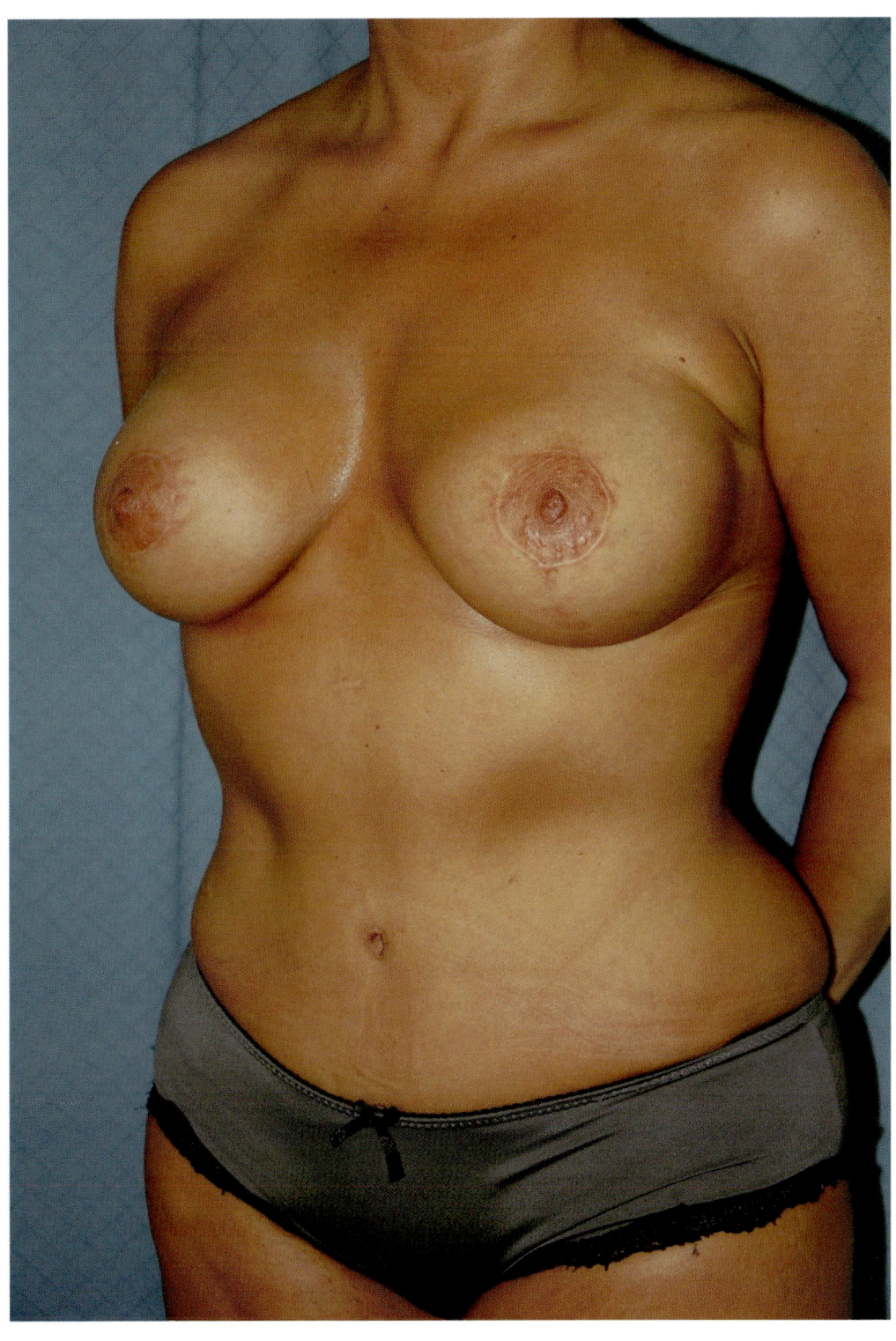

Front view

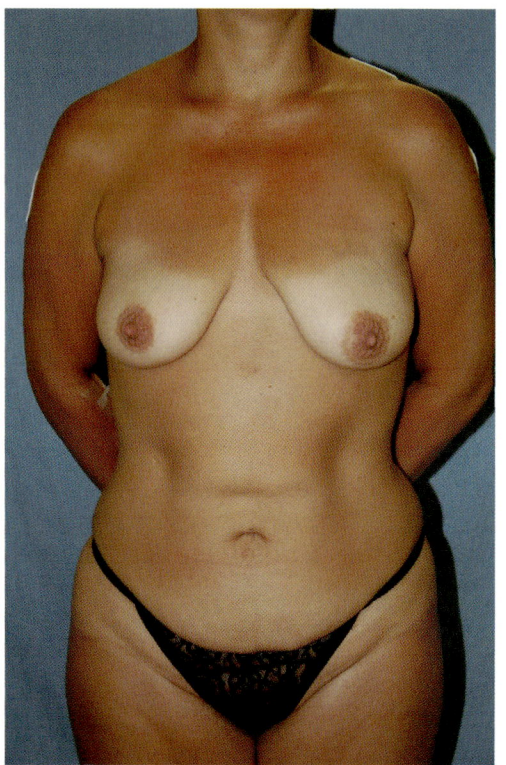
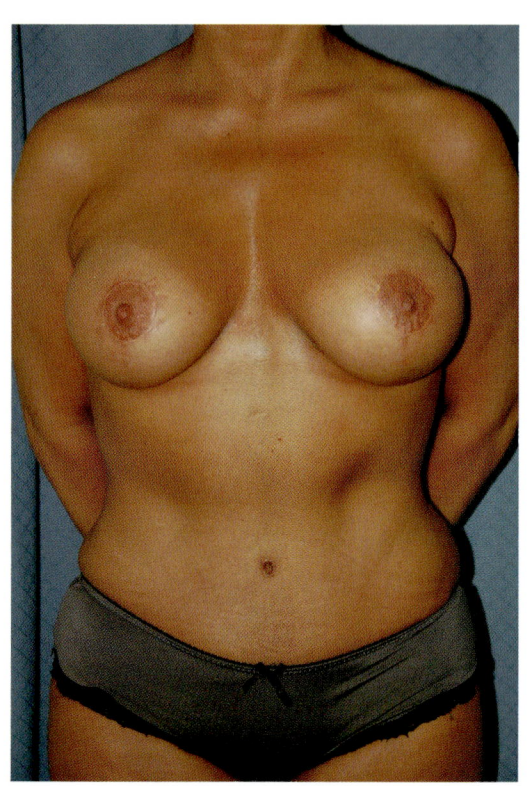

Side view

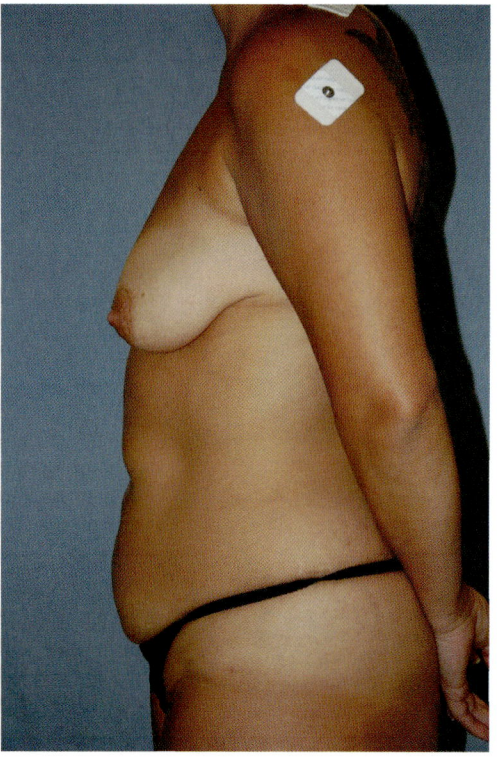
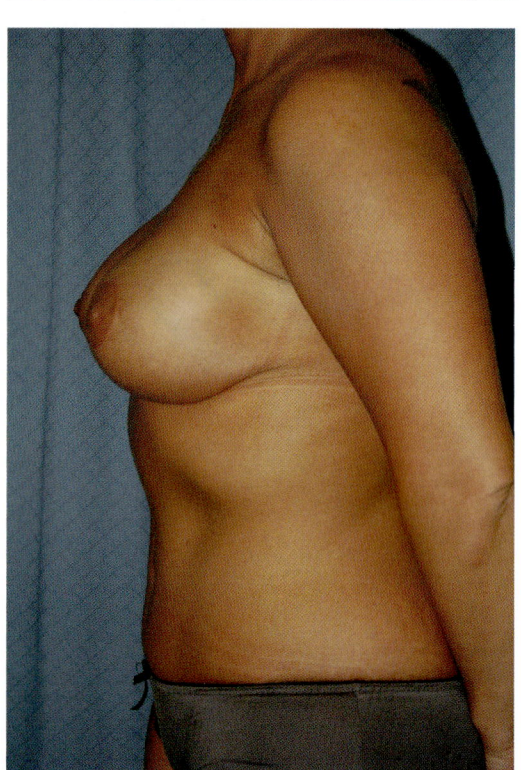

# Mommy Makeover Case 2

Angle view

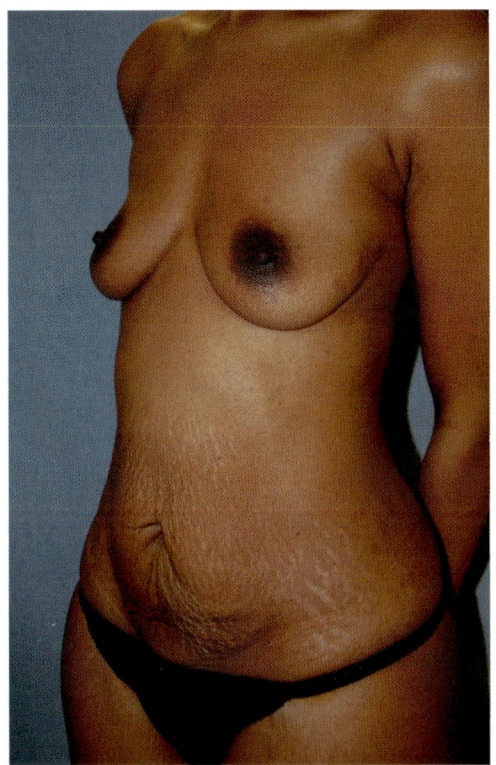 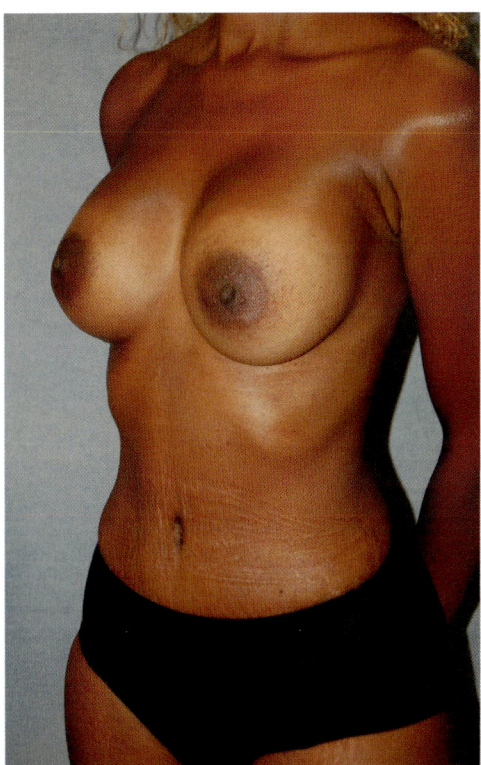

Side view

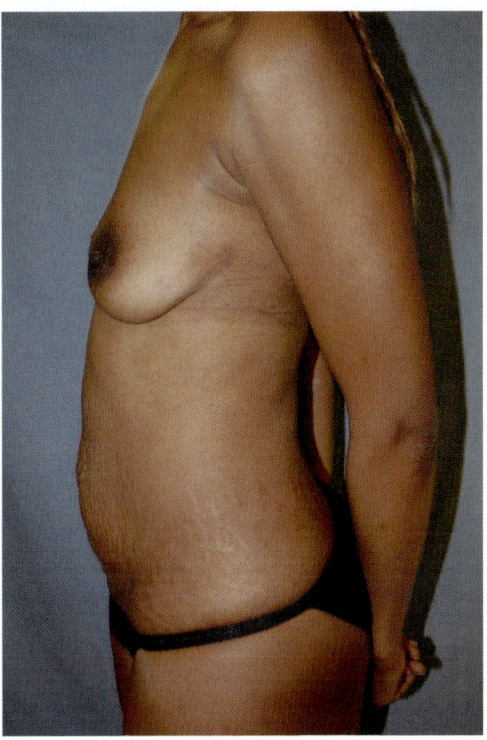 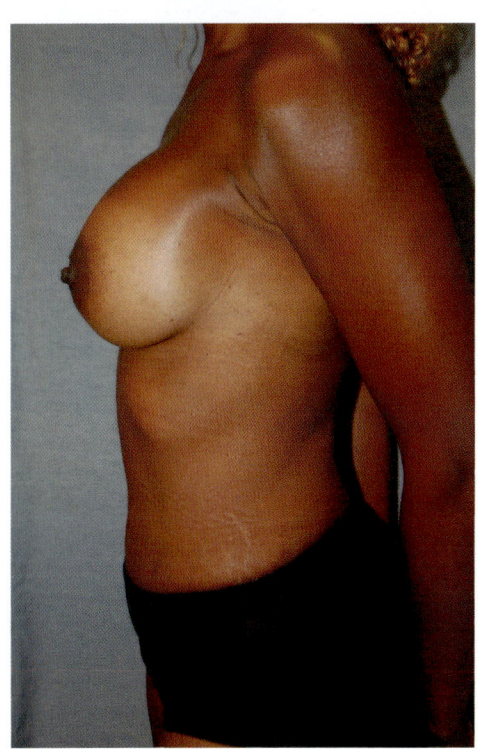

Front view

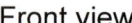

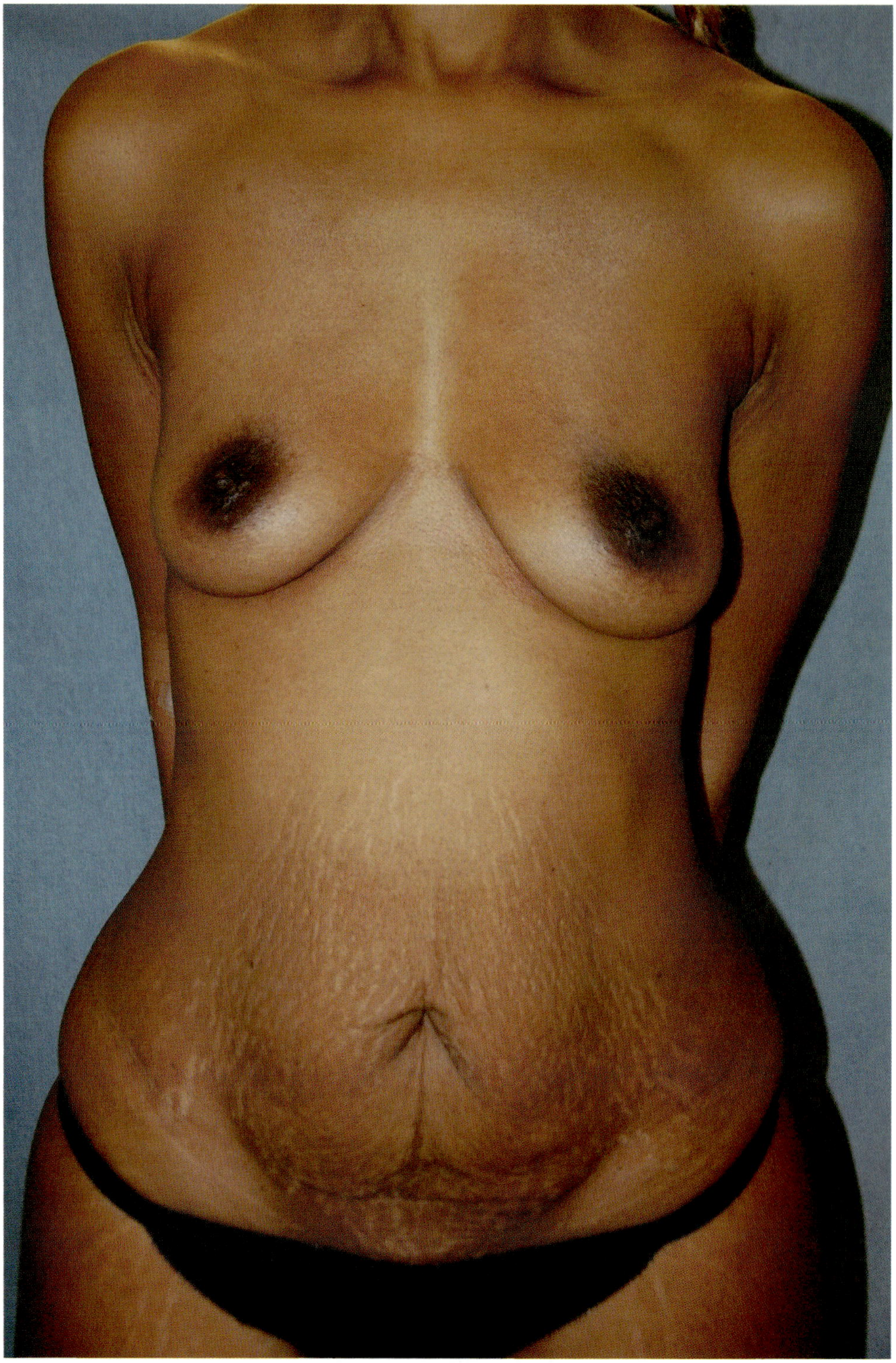

Front view

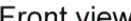

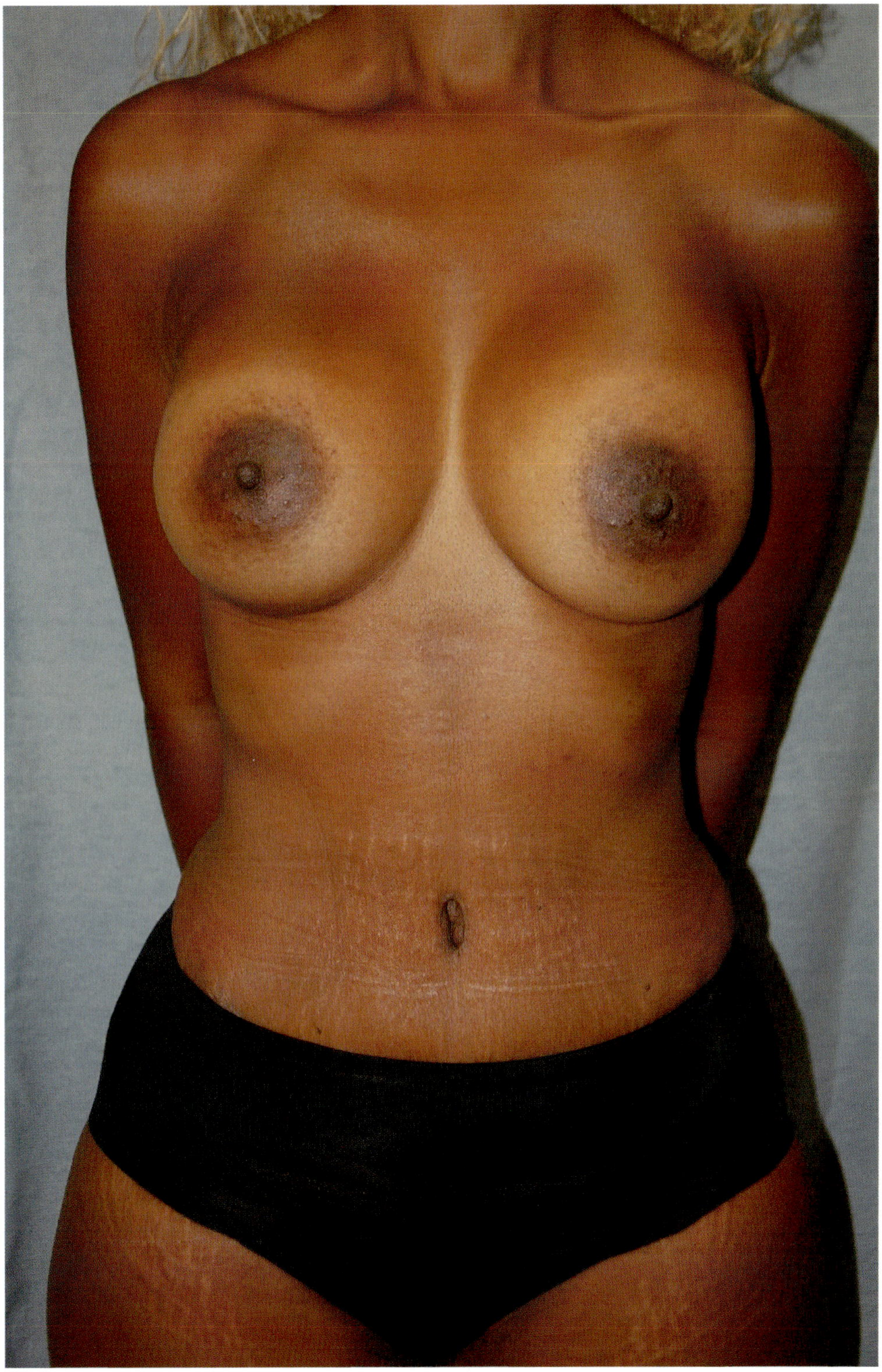

## Mommy Makeover Case 3

Side view

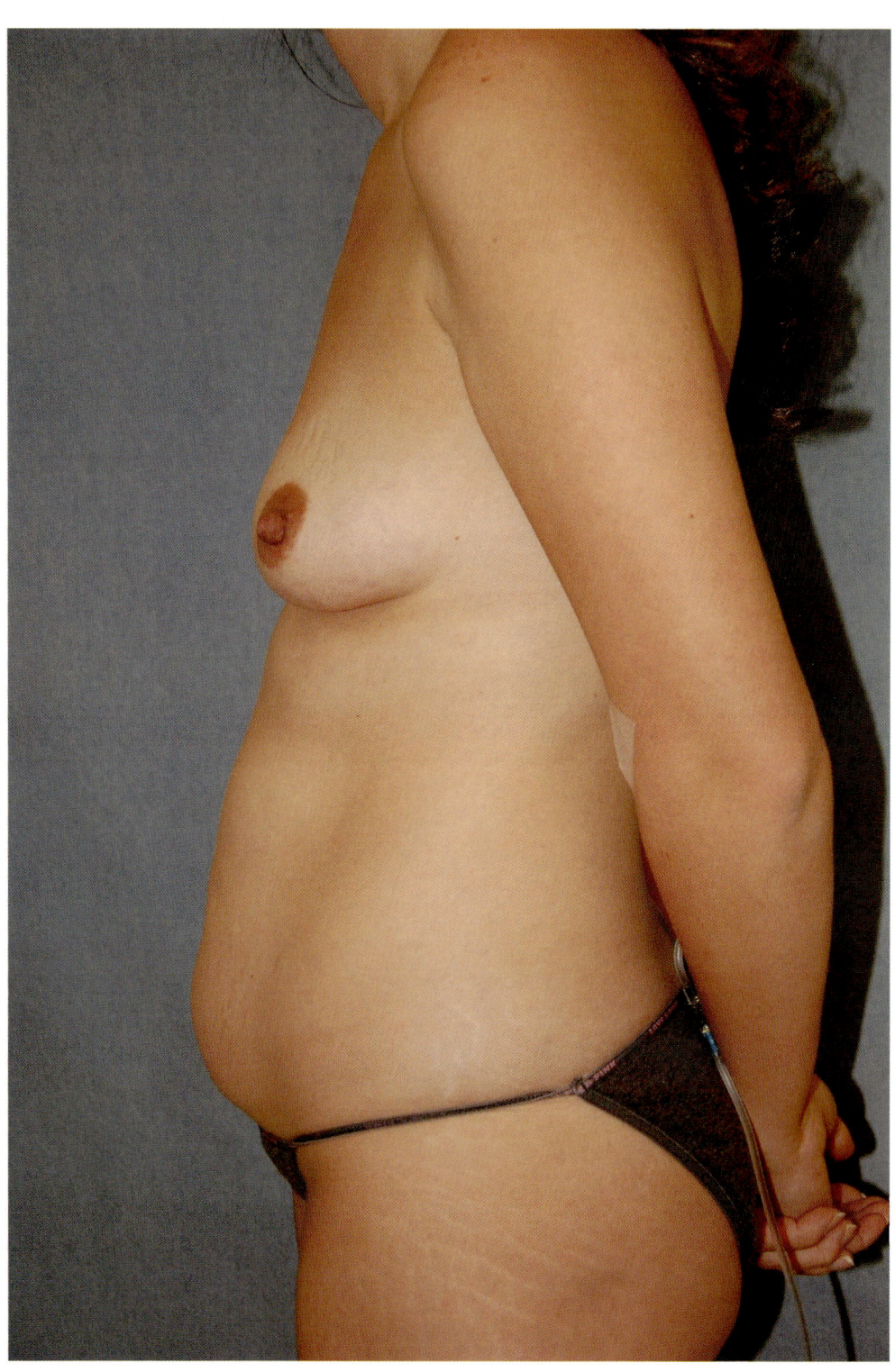

Side view

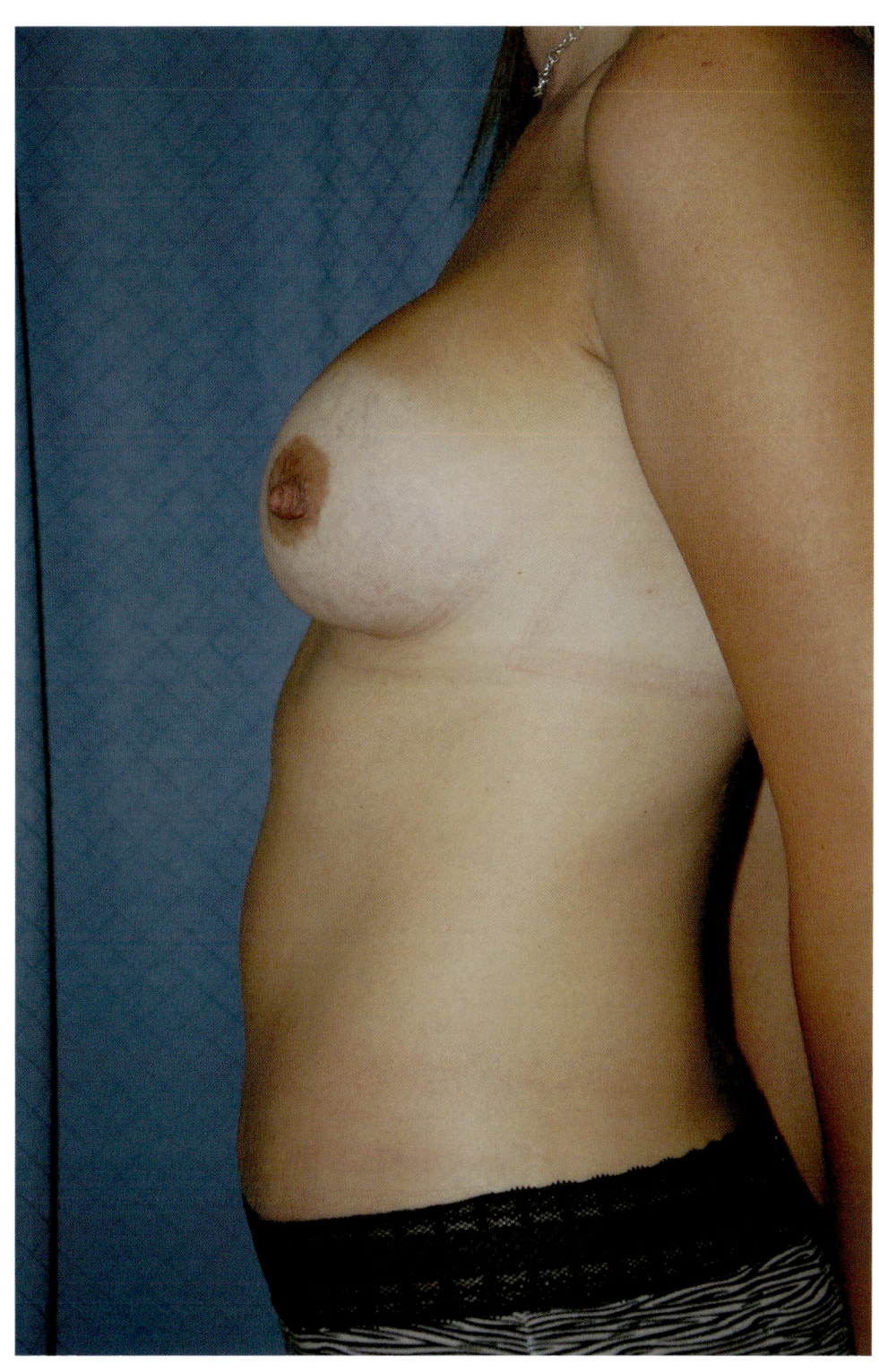

Front view

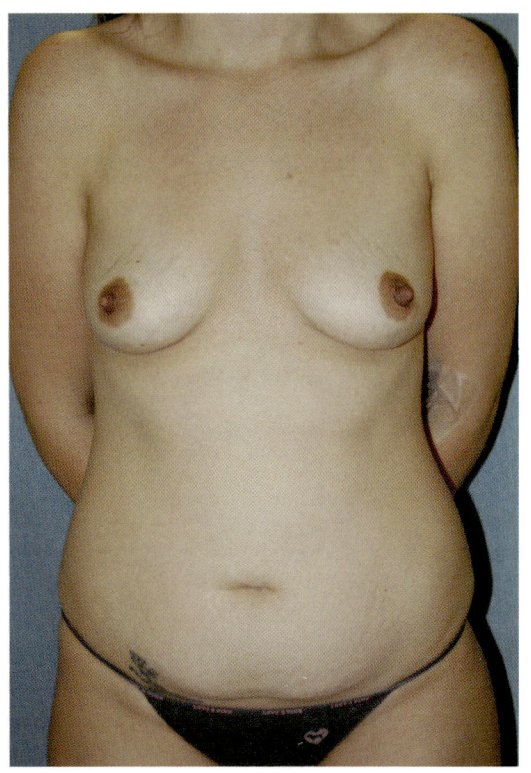 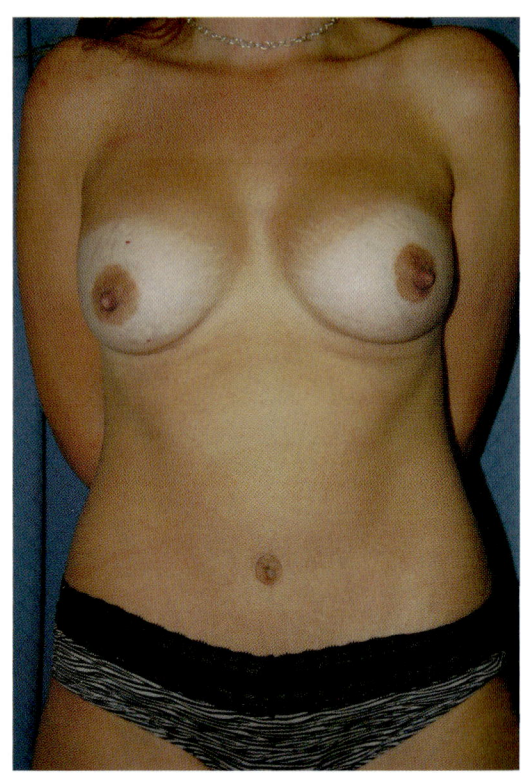

Angle view

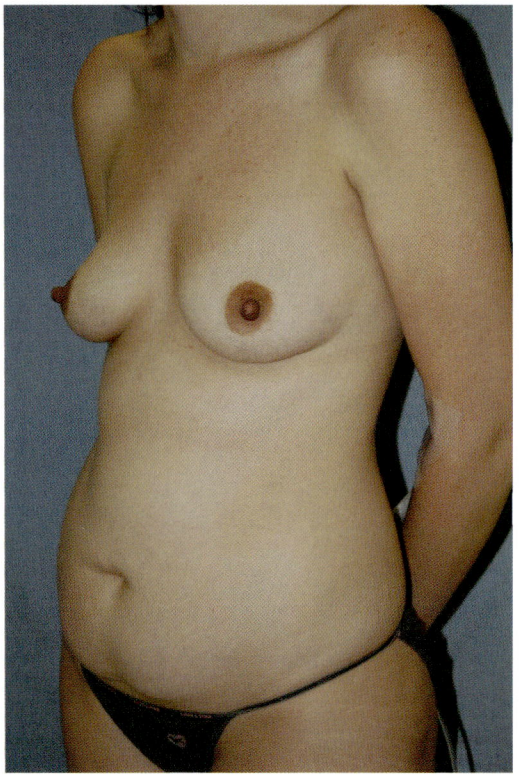 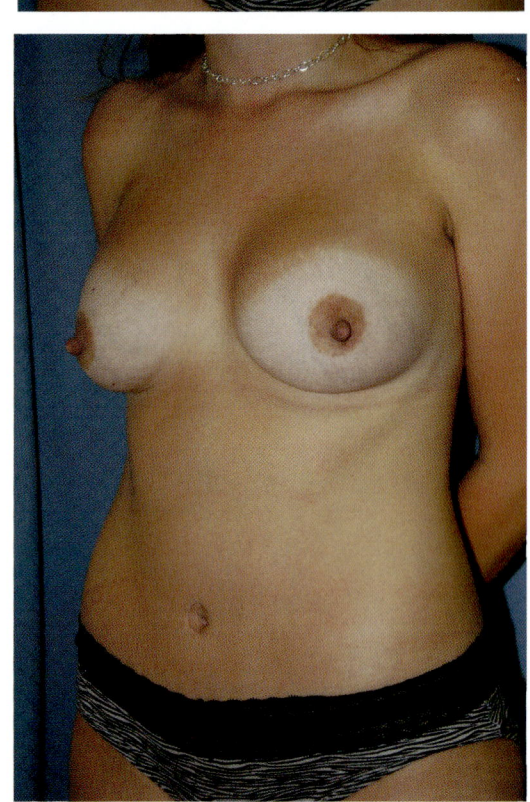

# Mommy Makeover Case 4

Front view

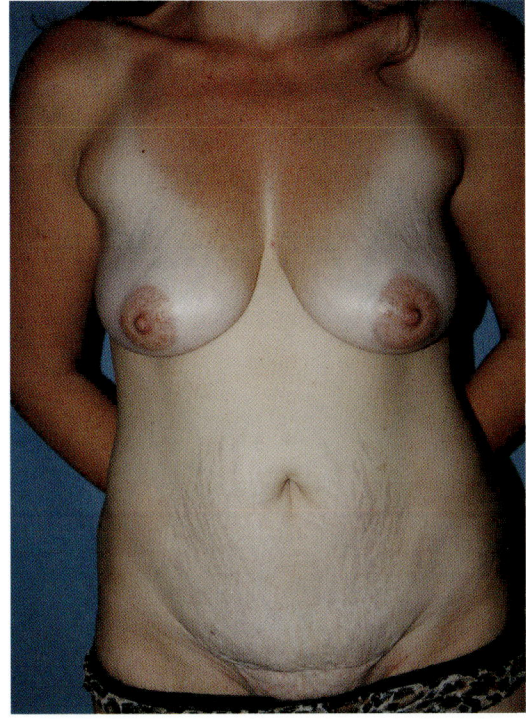 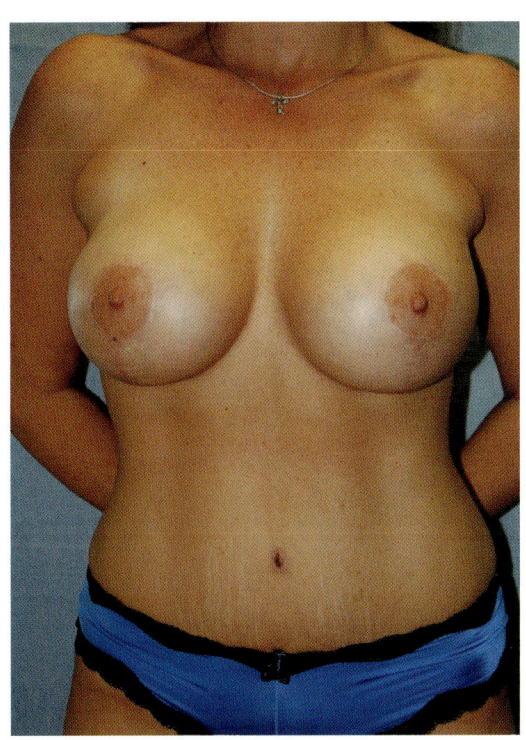

Side view

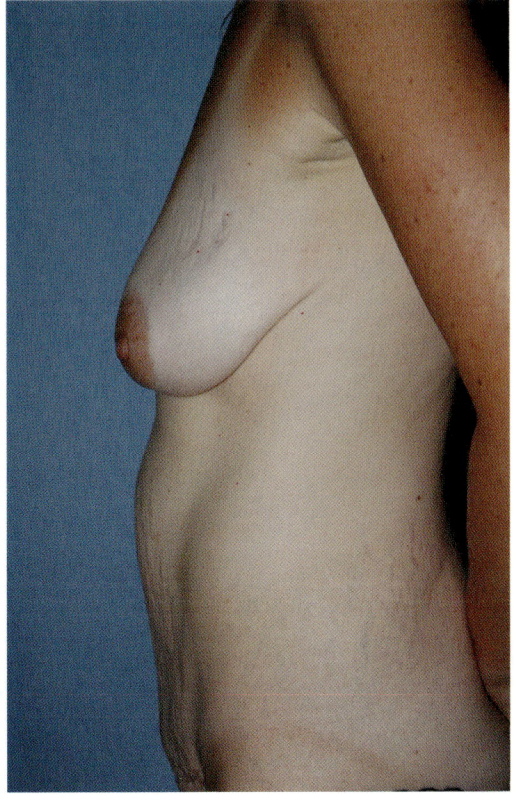 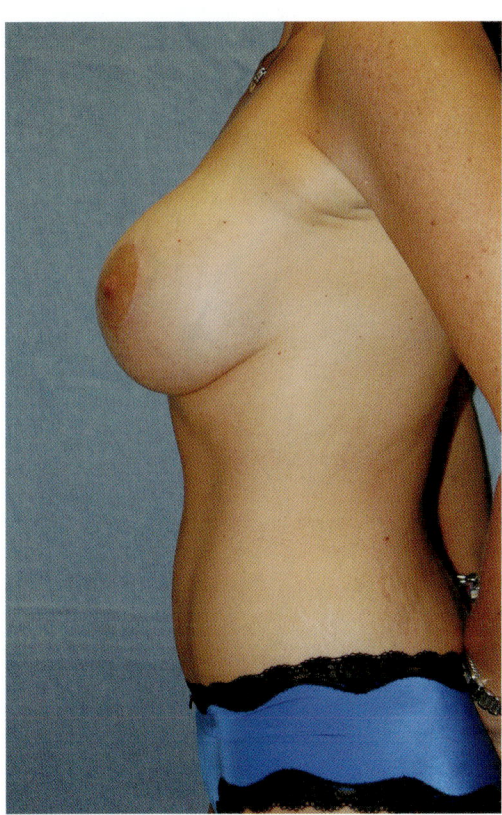

Angle view

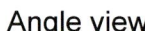

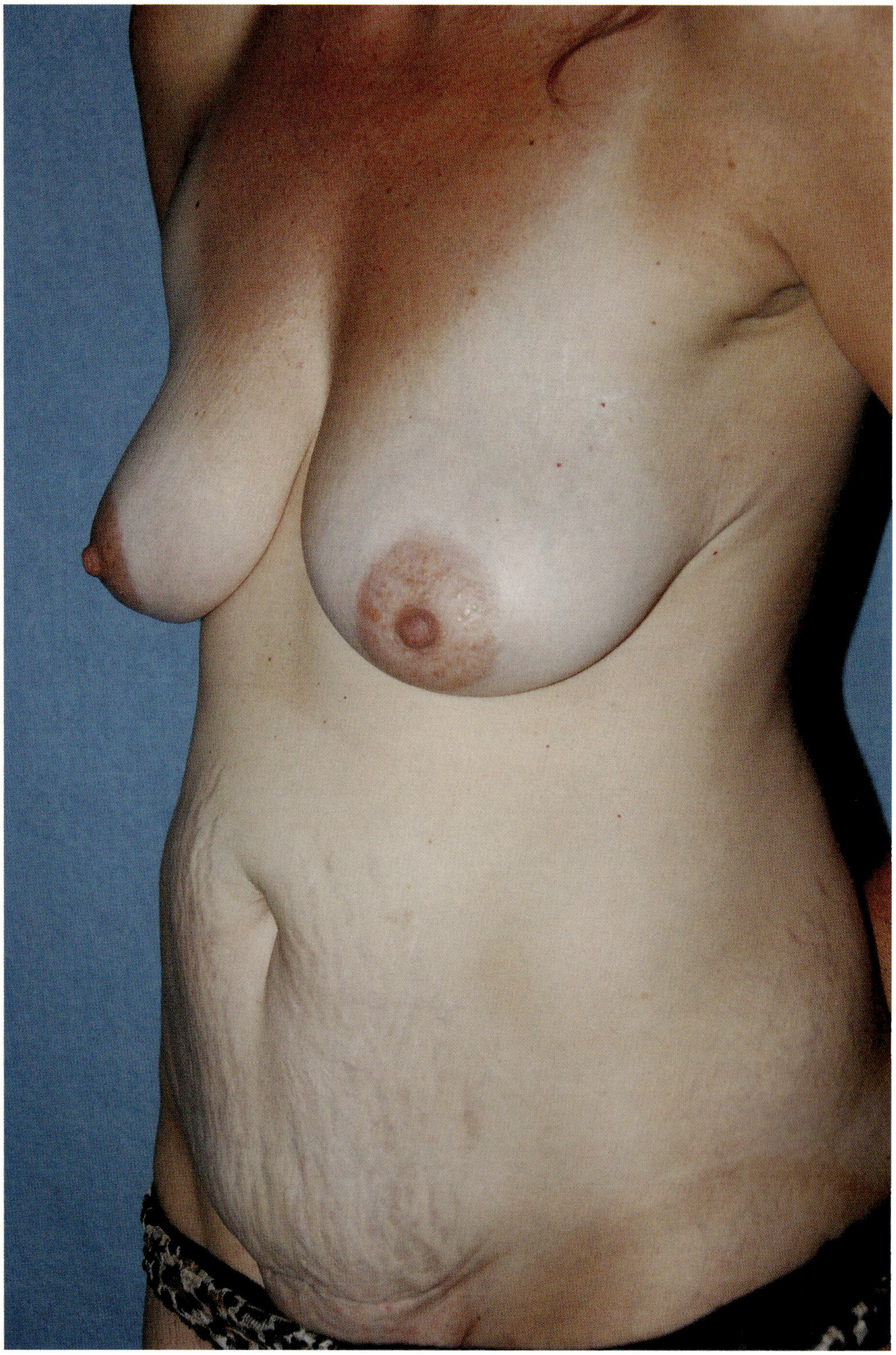

Angle view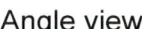

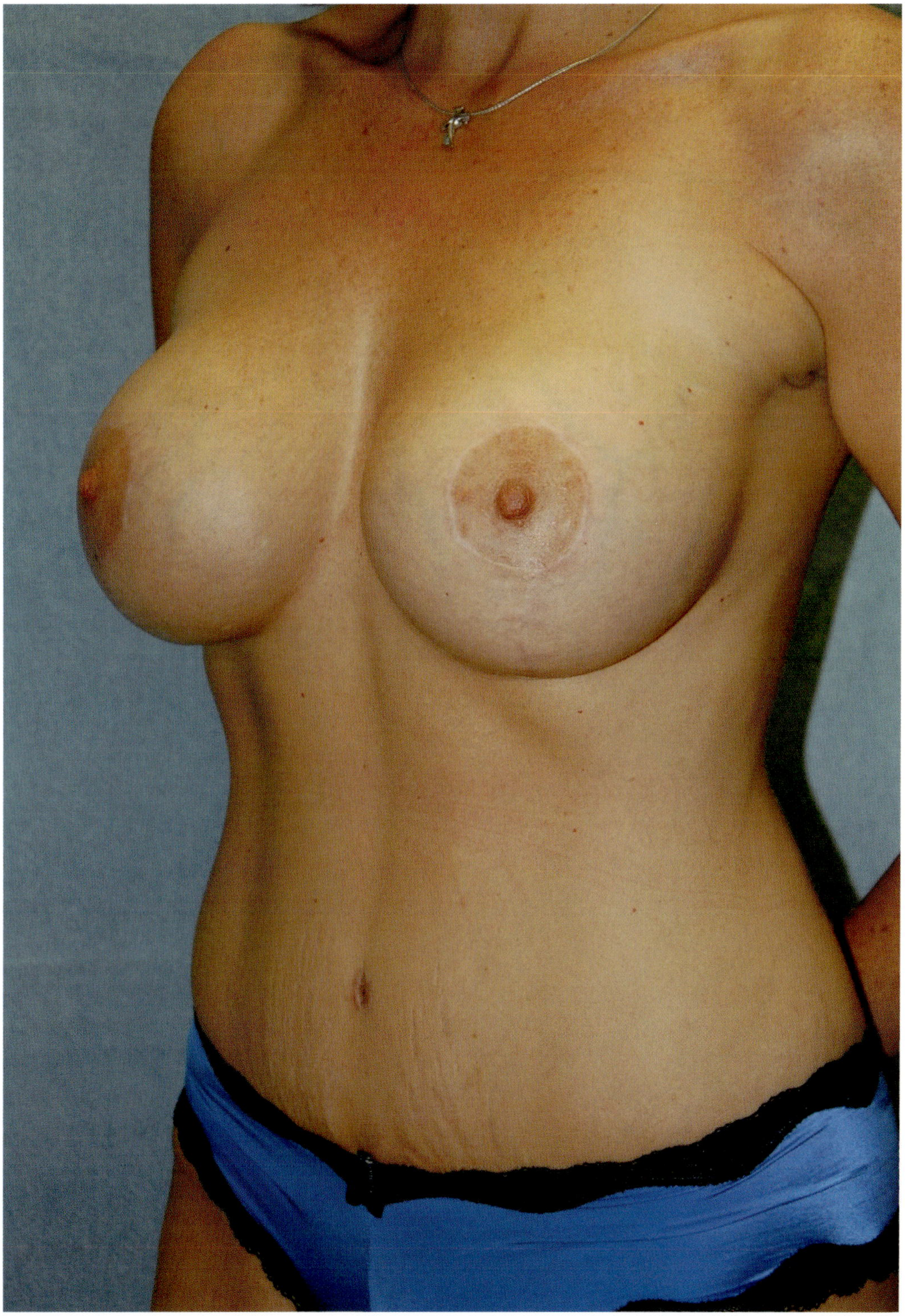

# Mommy Makeover Case 5

Angle view

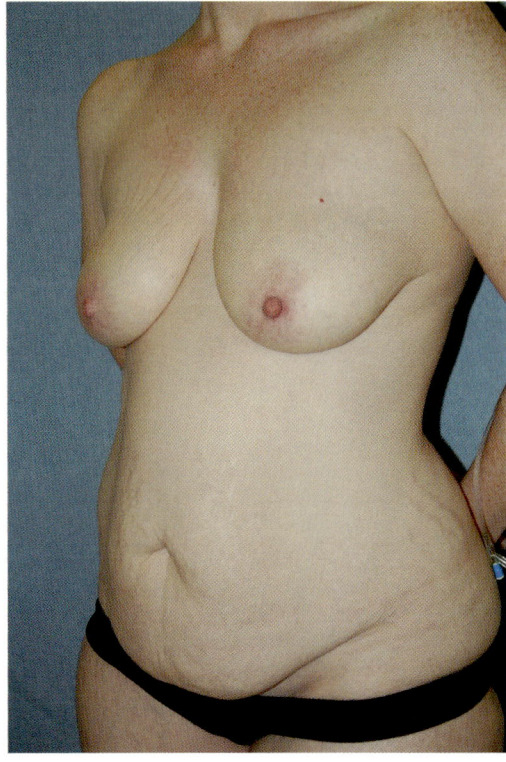 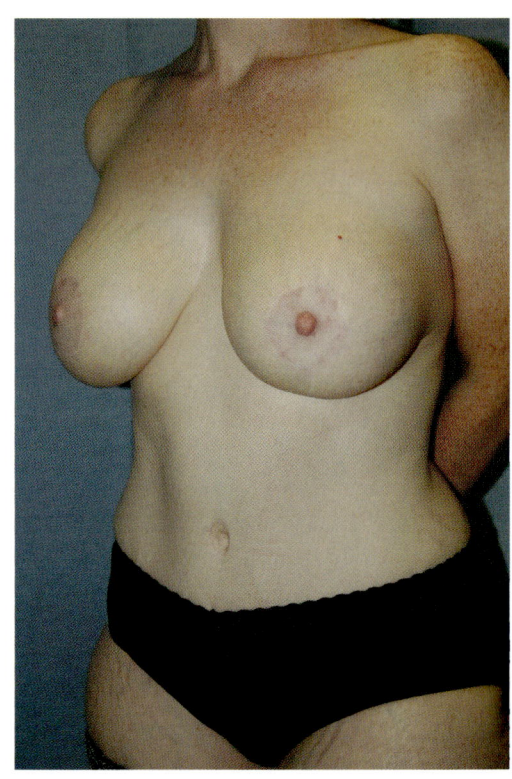

Angle view

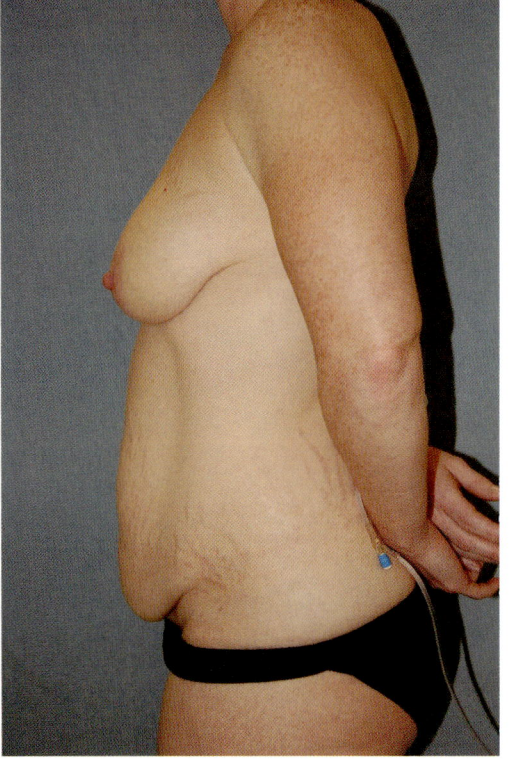 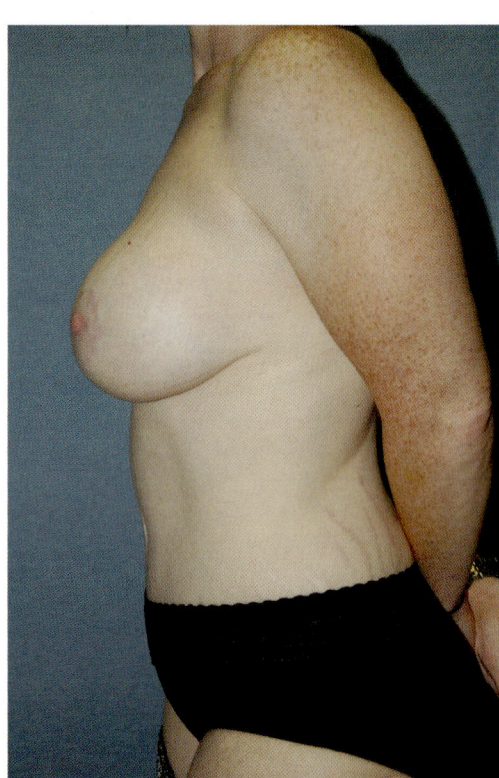

# Tummy Tuck Case 1

Angle view

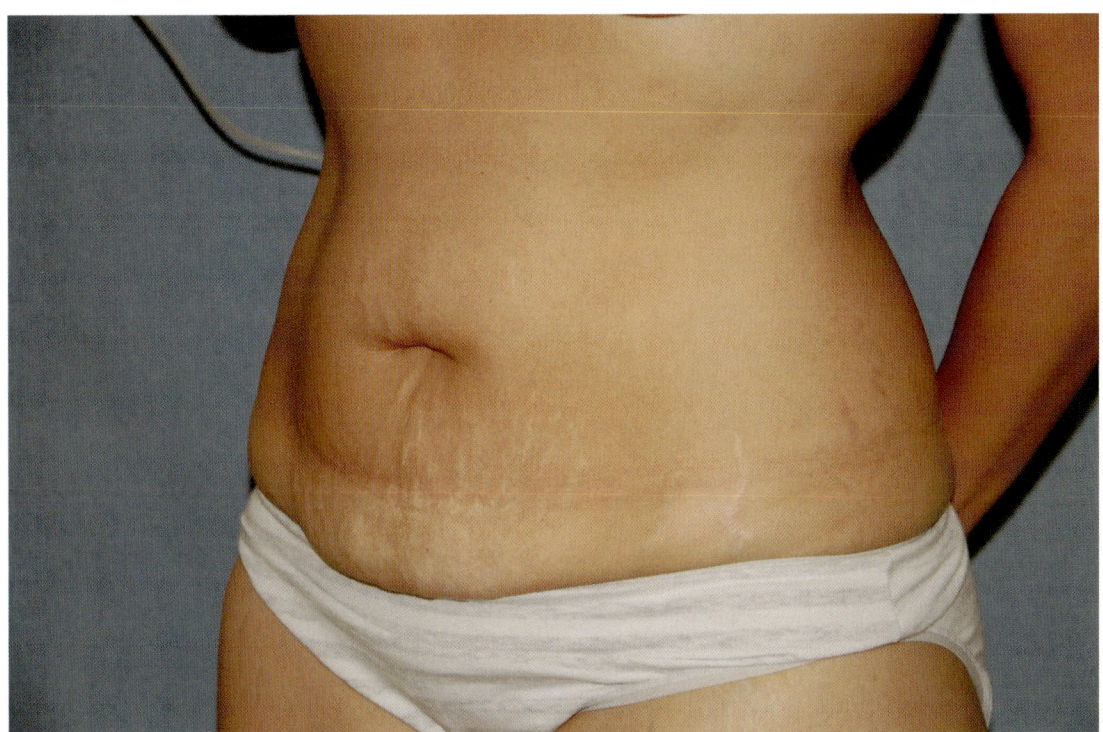

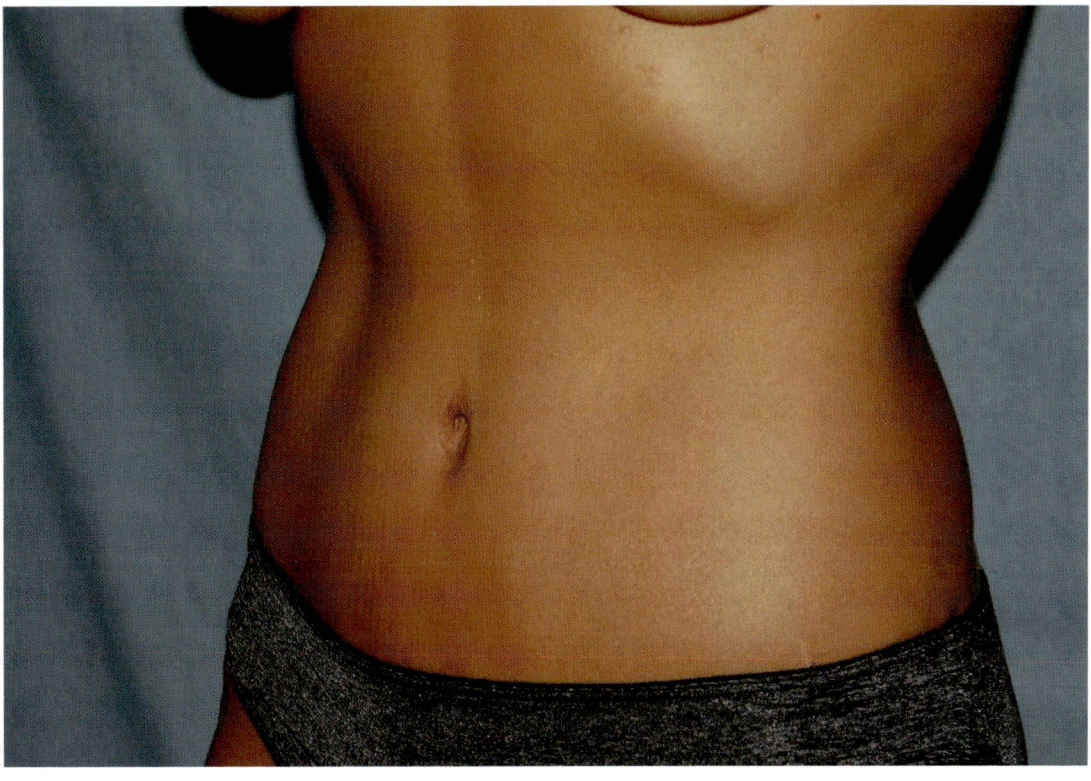

Front and side view

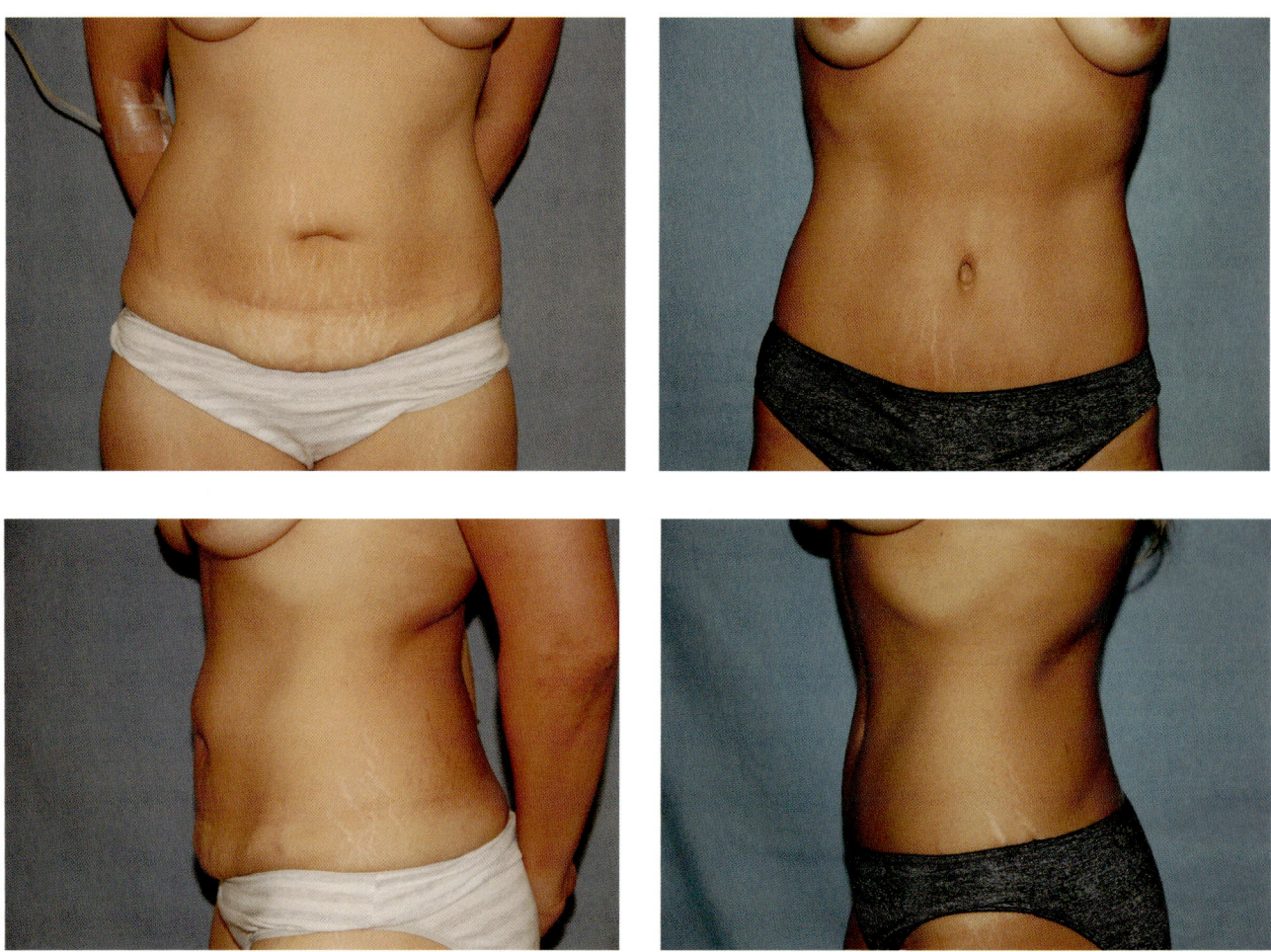

# Tummy Tuck Case 2

Front, angle, and side view

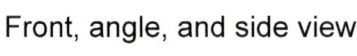

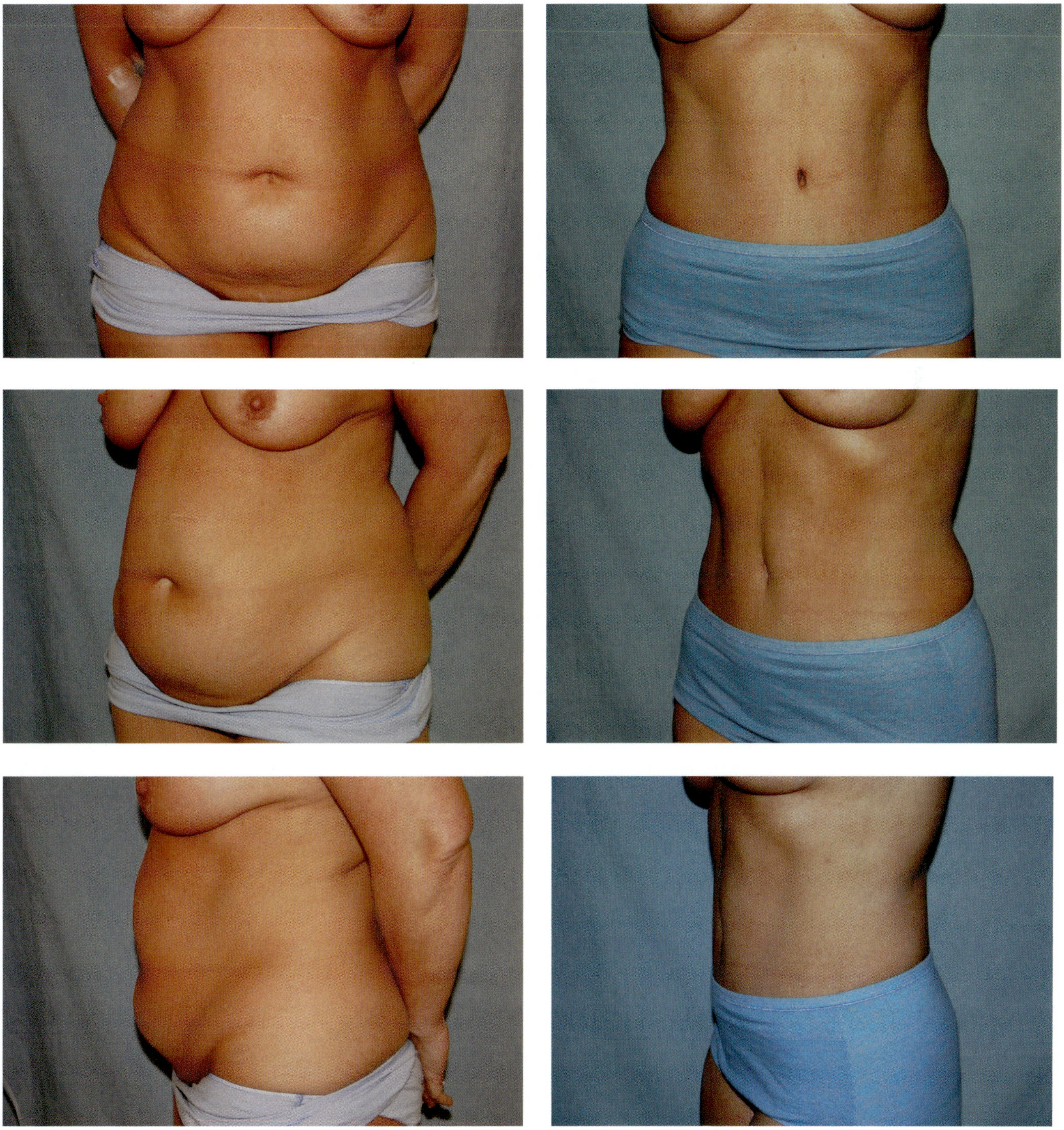

# Tummy Tuck Case 3

Front, angle, and side view

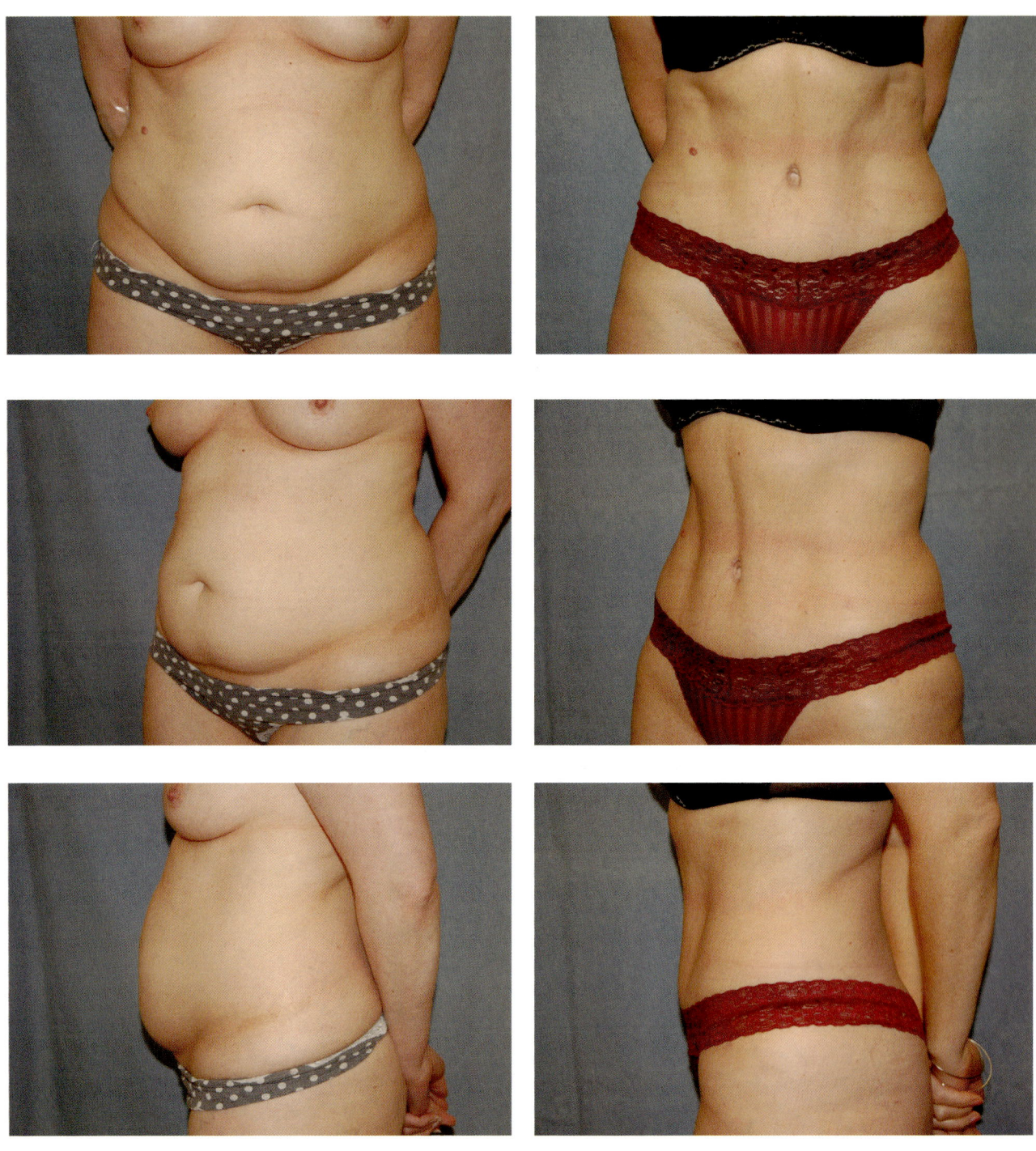

# Tummy Tuck Case 4

Front, angle, and side view

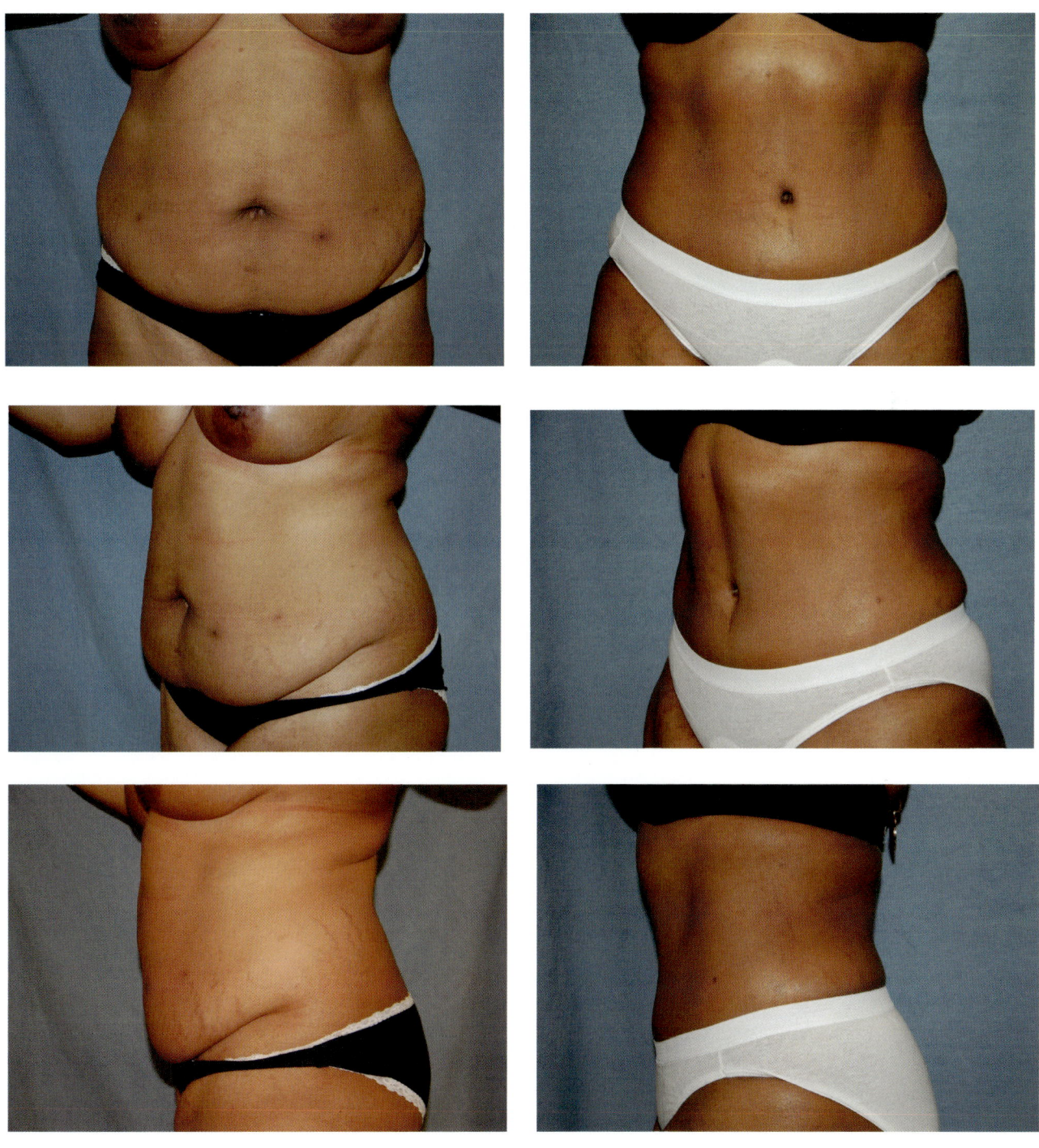

# Face, Neck, and Eyelid Rejuvenation Case 1

Angle view

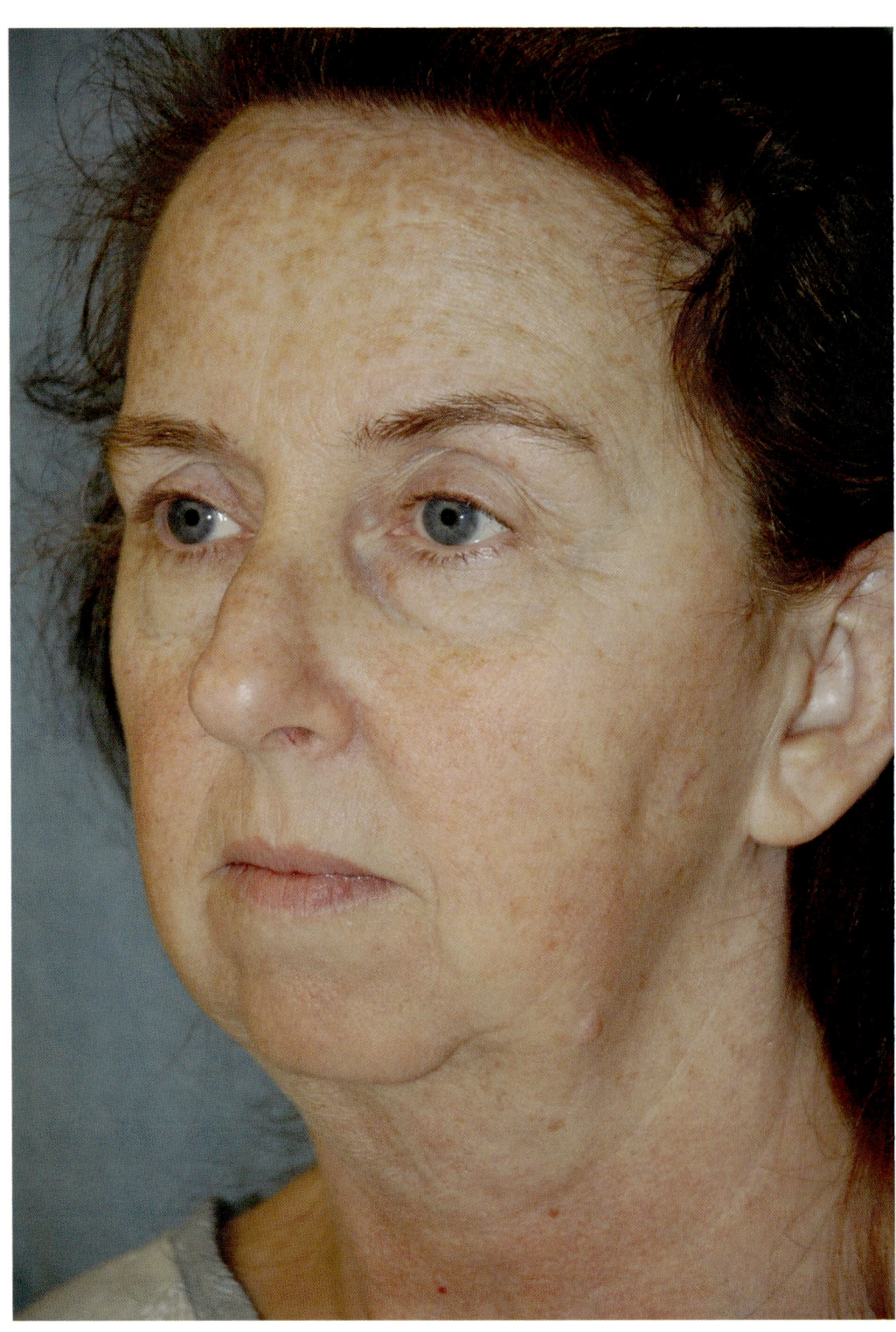

Angle view

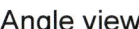

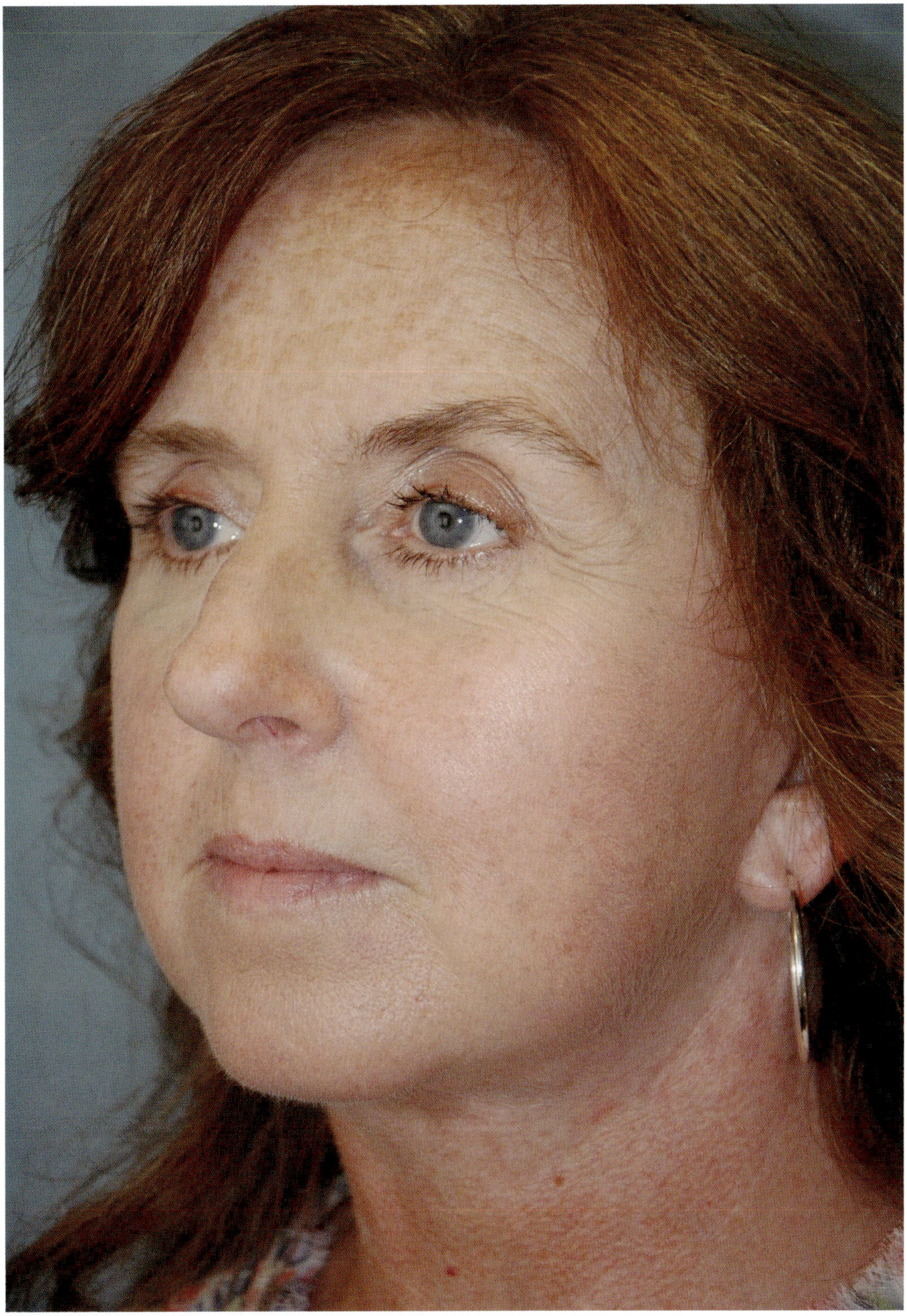

Front view

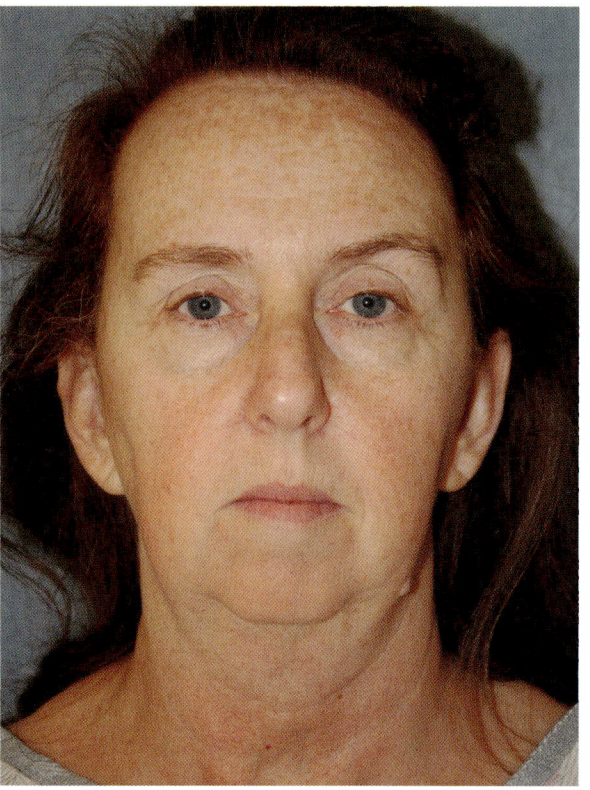
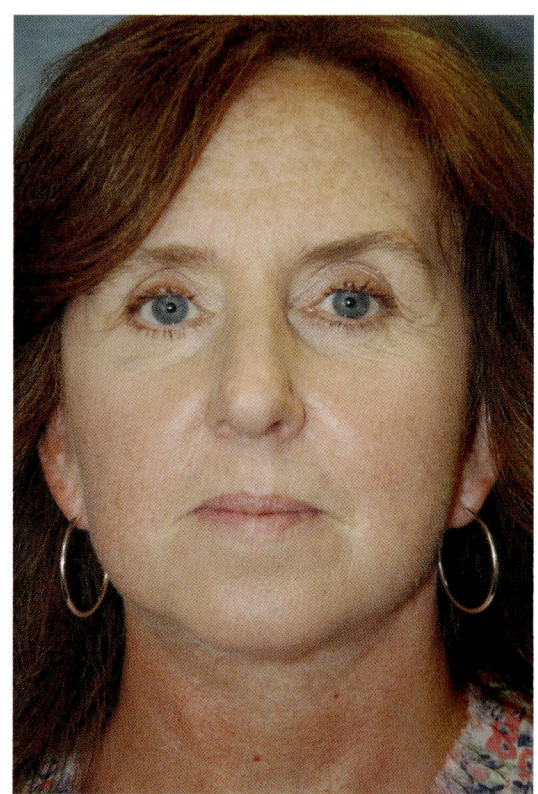

Side view

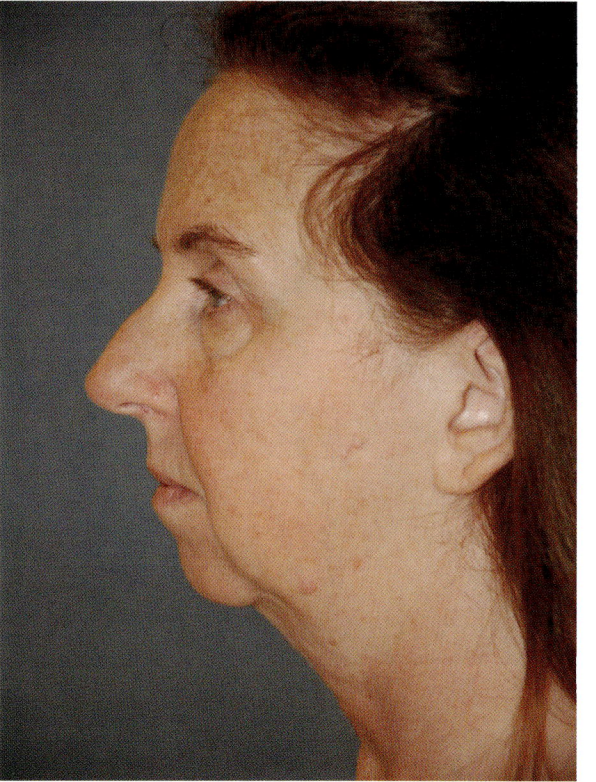
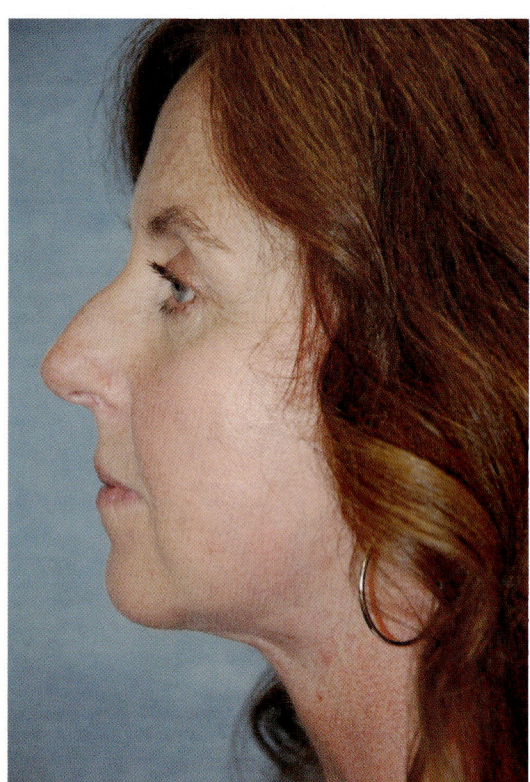

# Face, Neck, and Eyelid Rejuvenation Case 2

Front view

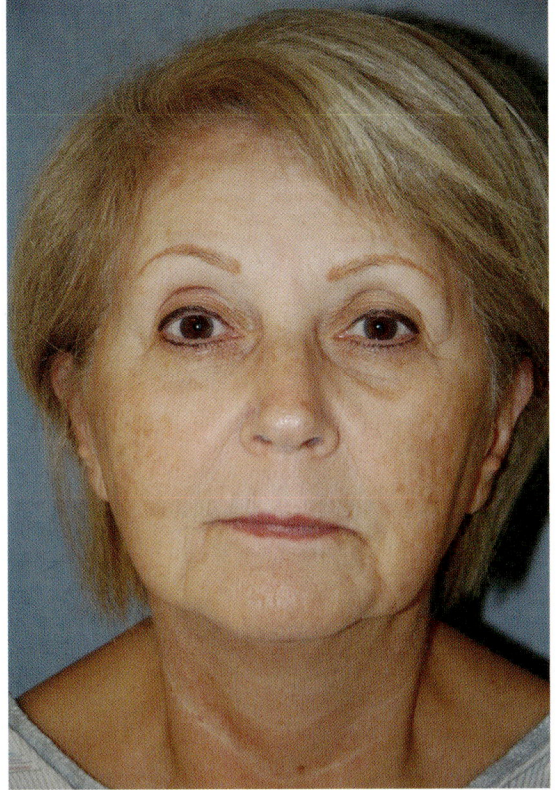 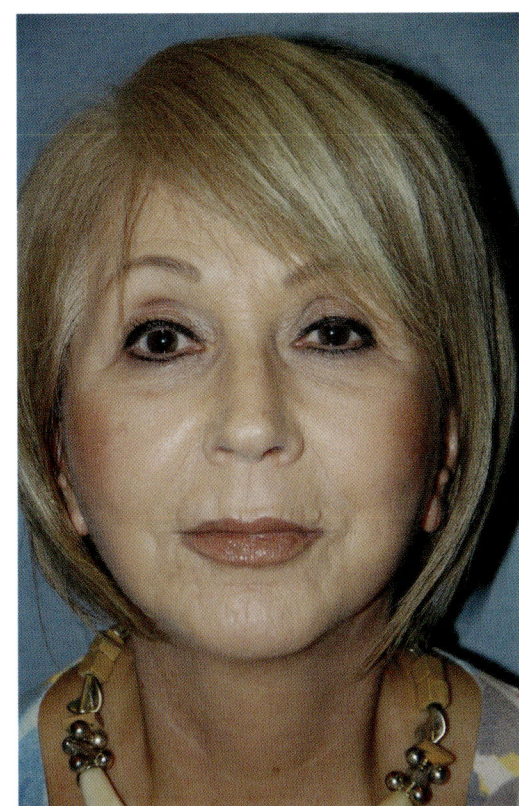

Front view

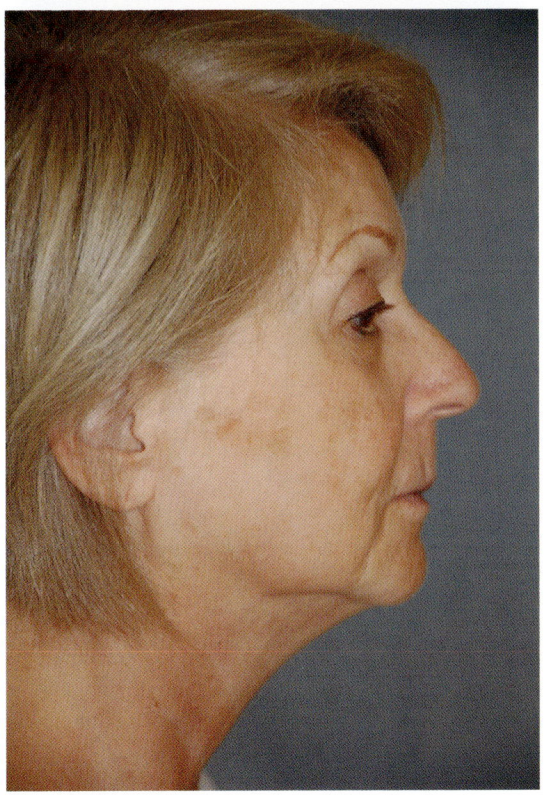 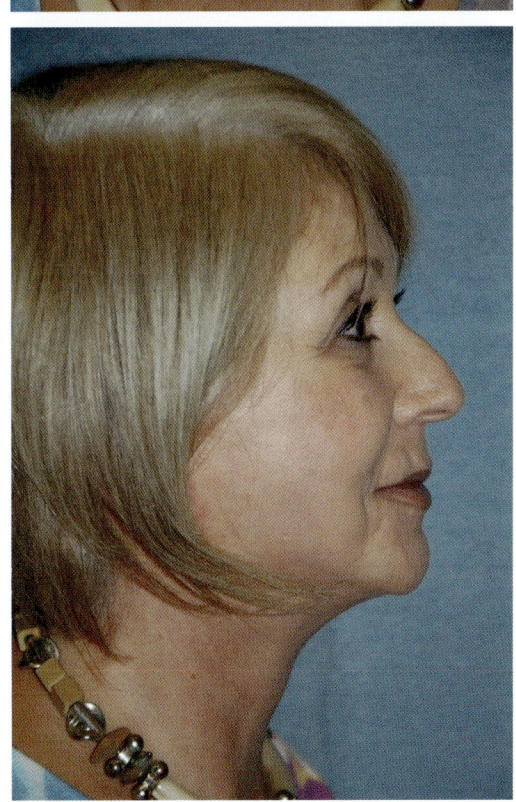

Angle view

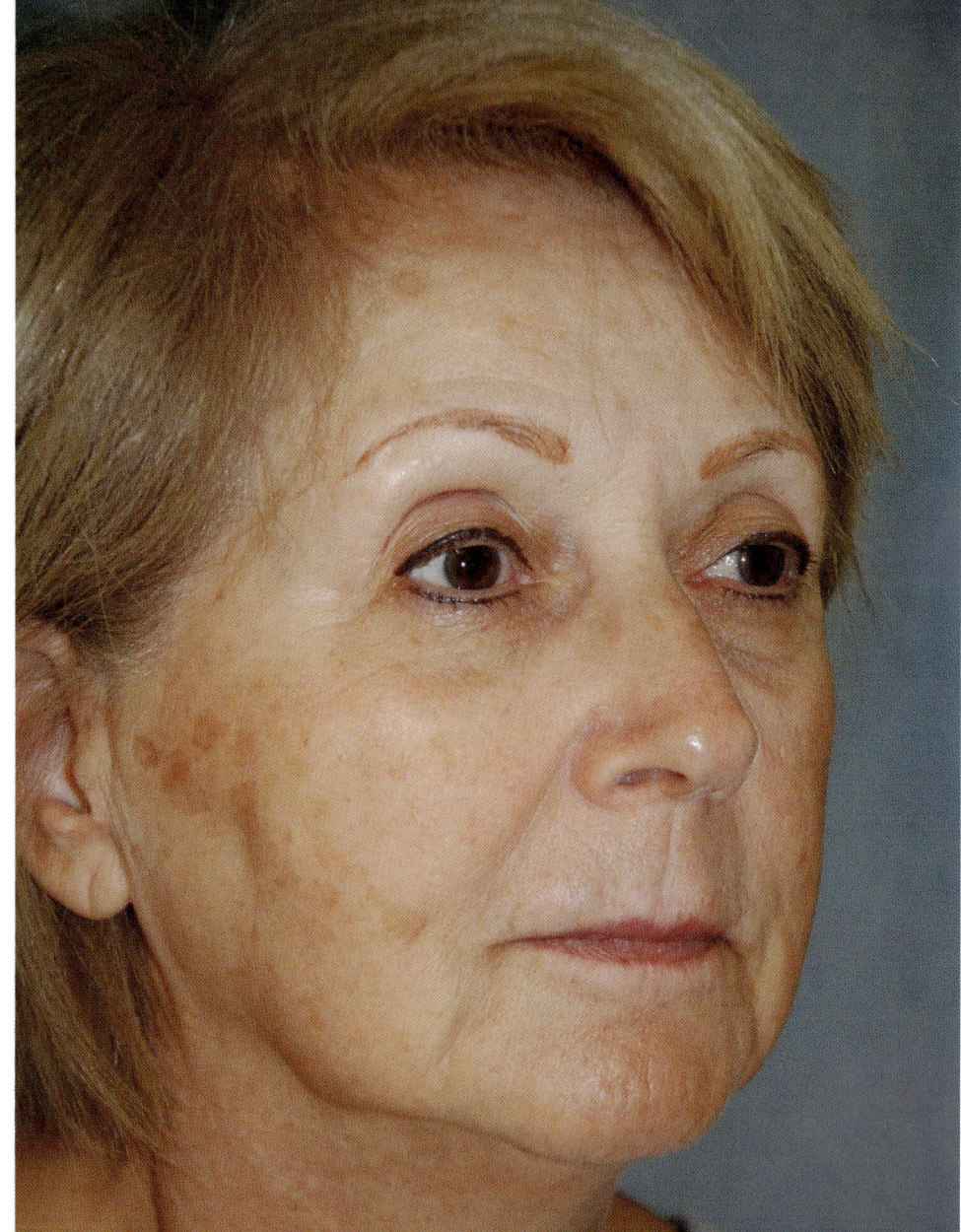

Angle view

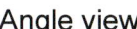

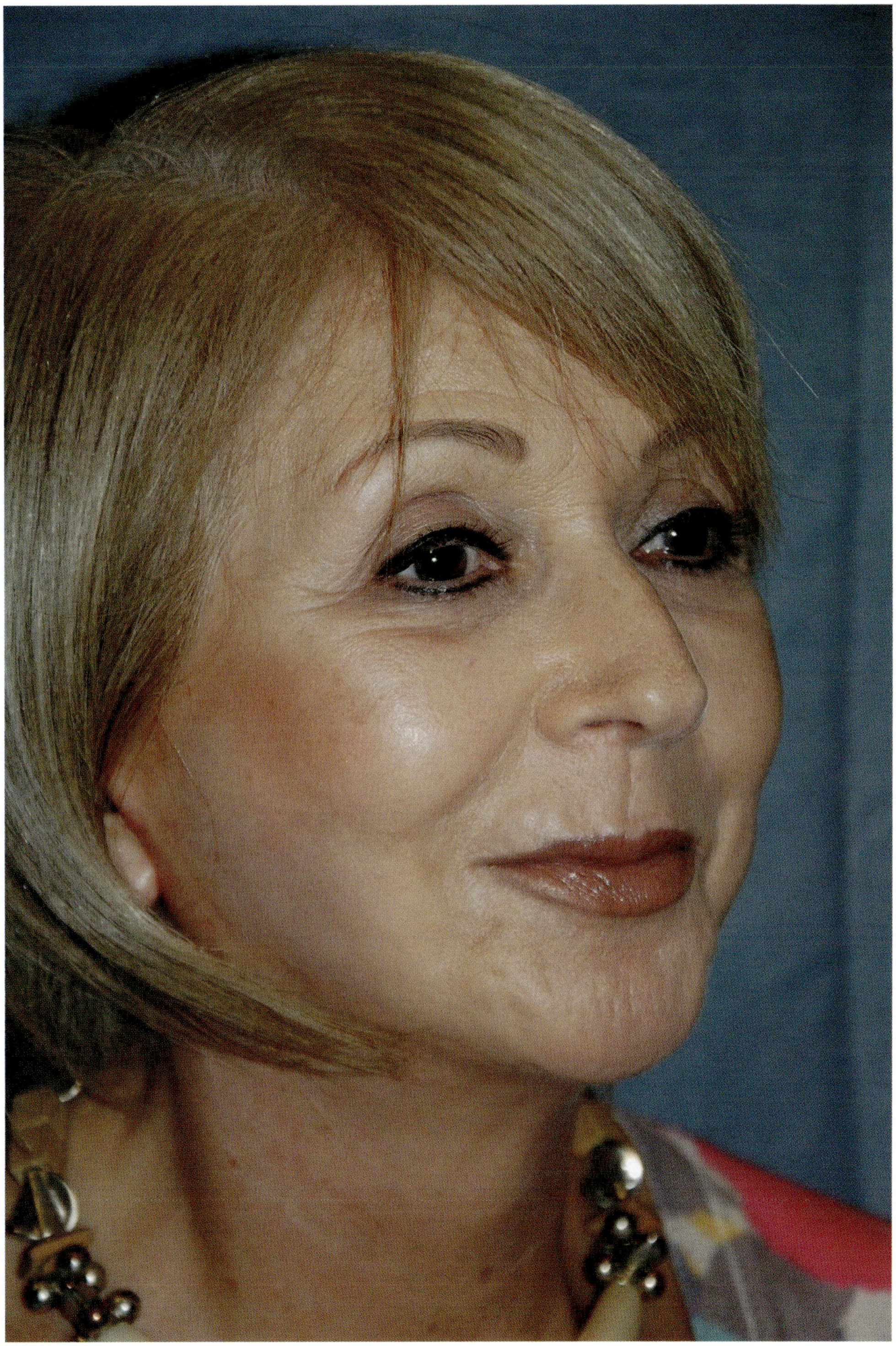

# Face, Neck, and Eyelid Rejuvenation Case 3

Side view

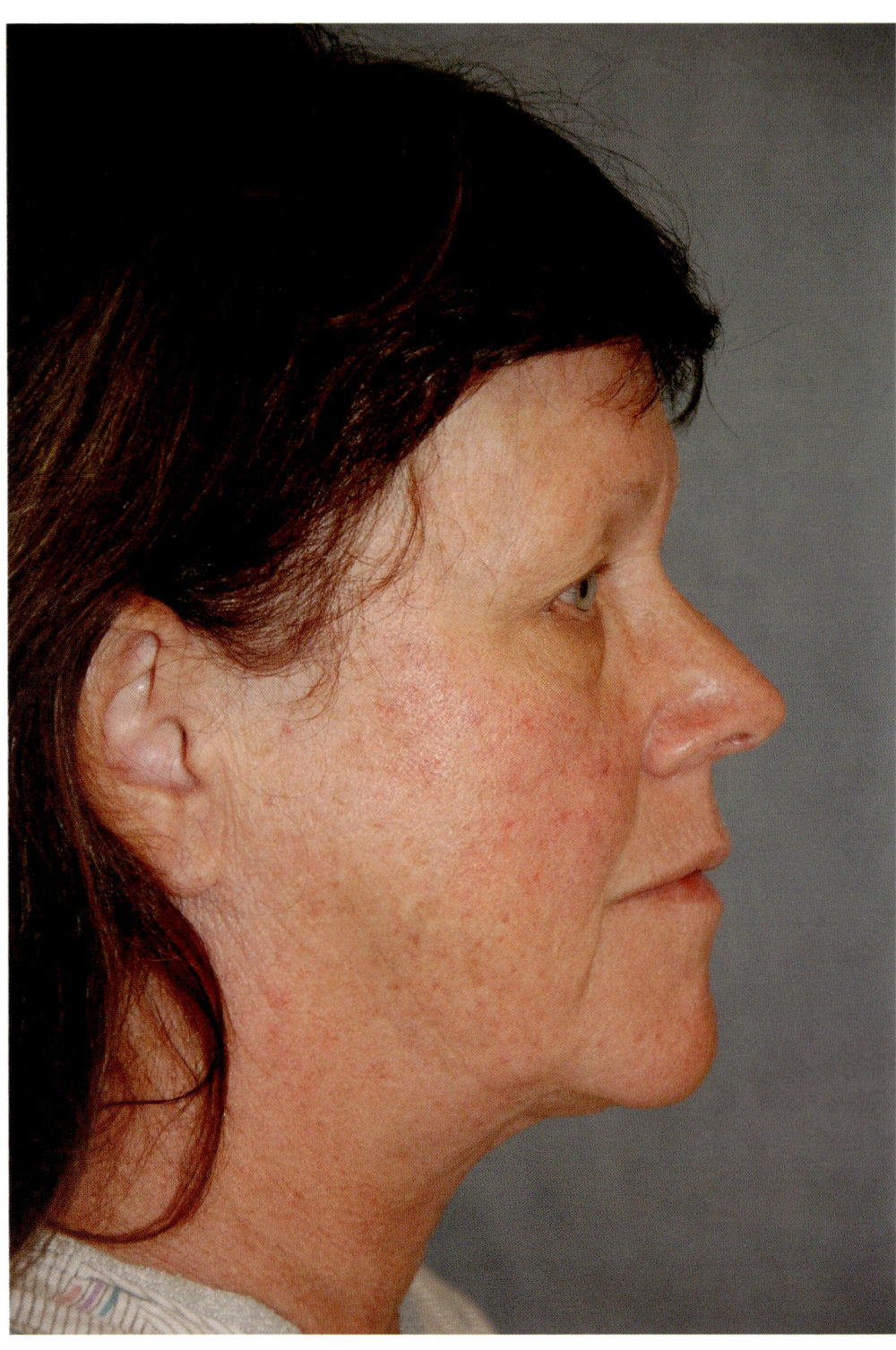

Side view

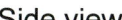

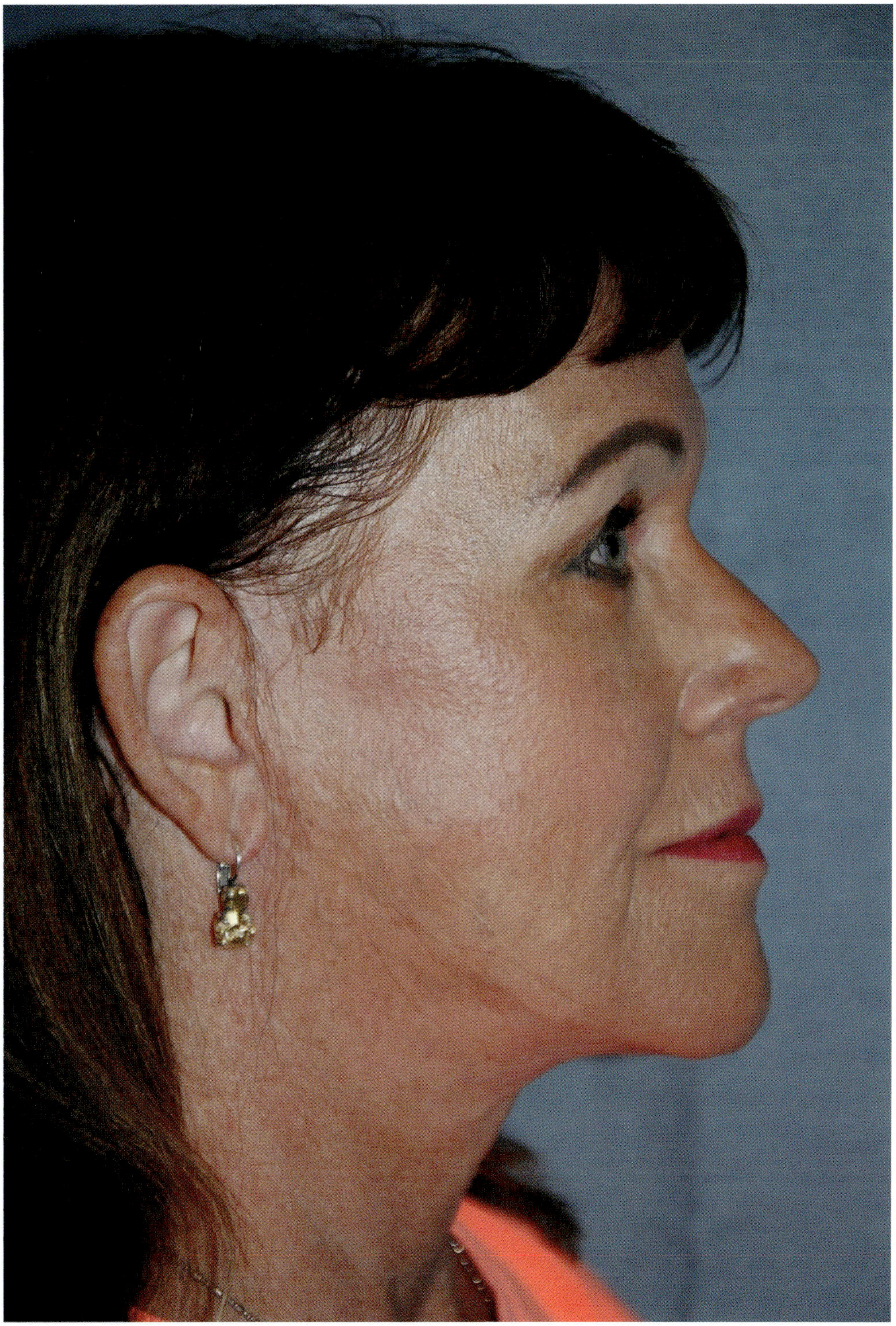

Front view

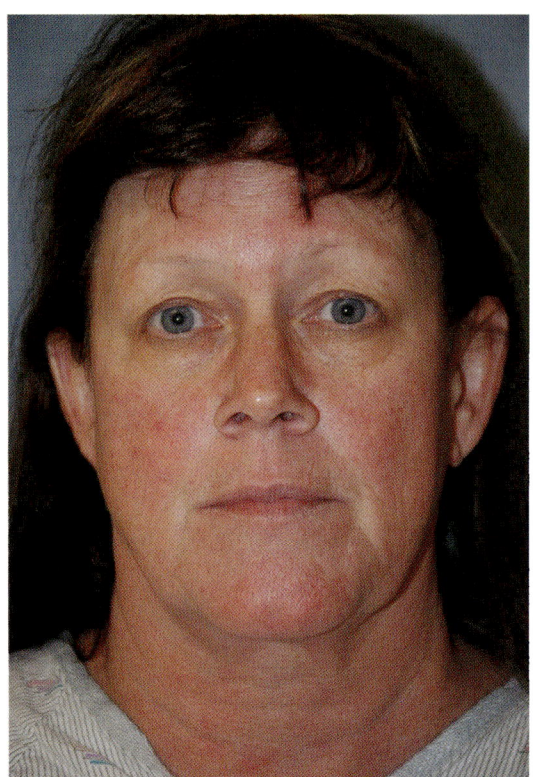 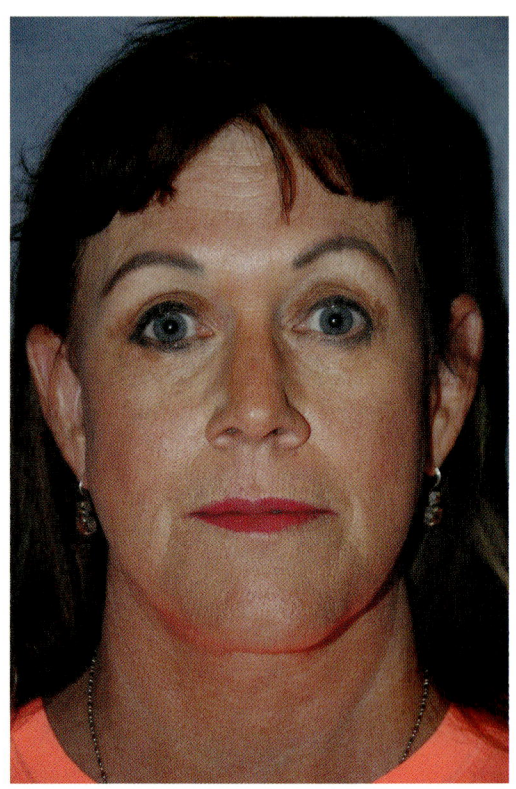

Angle view

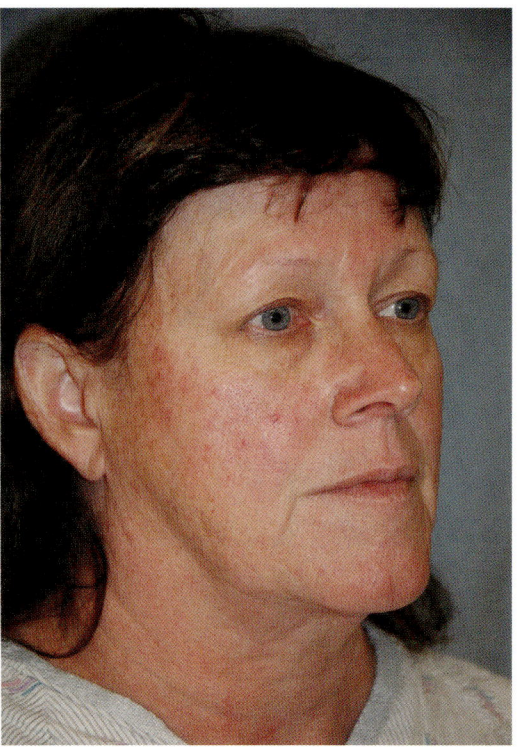 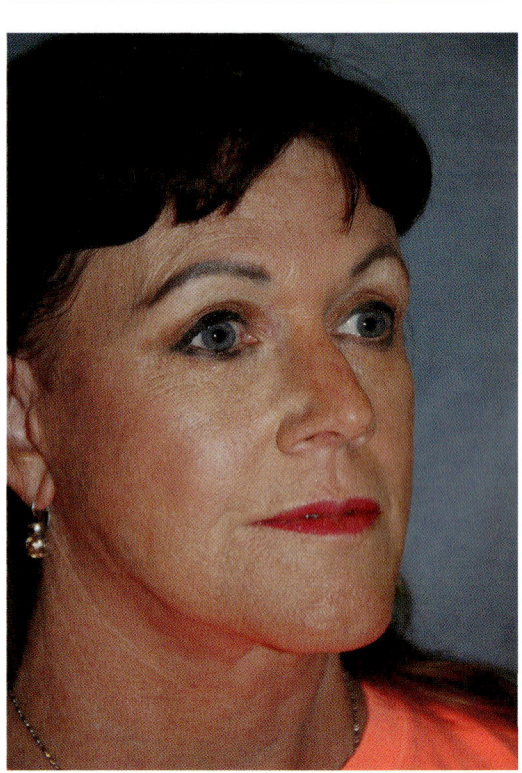

# Face, Neck, and Eyelid Rejuvenation Case 4

Front view

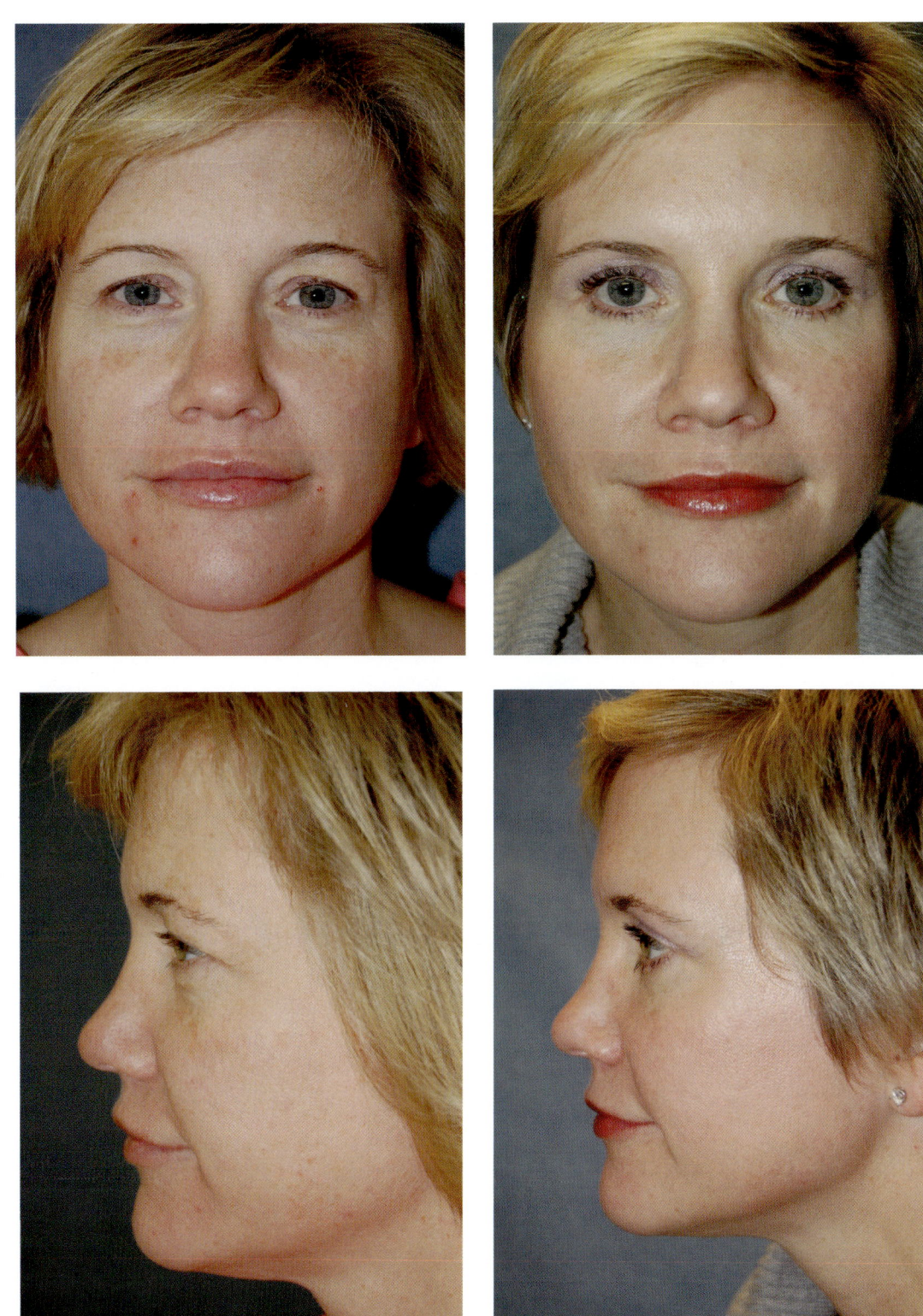

Angle view

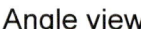

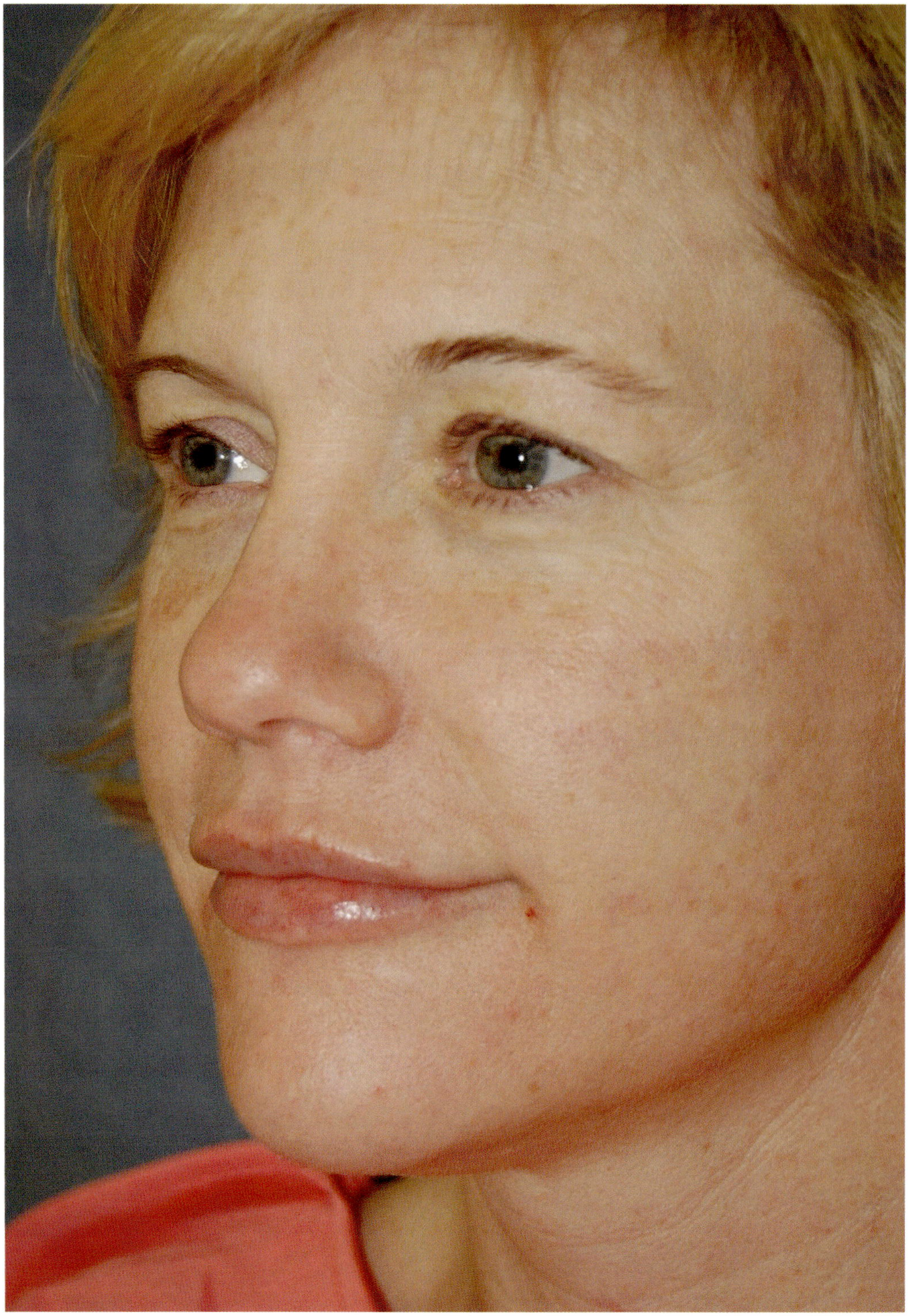

Angle view

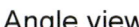

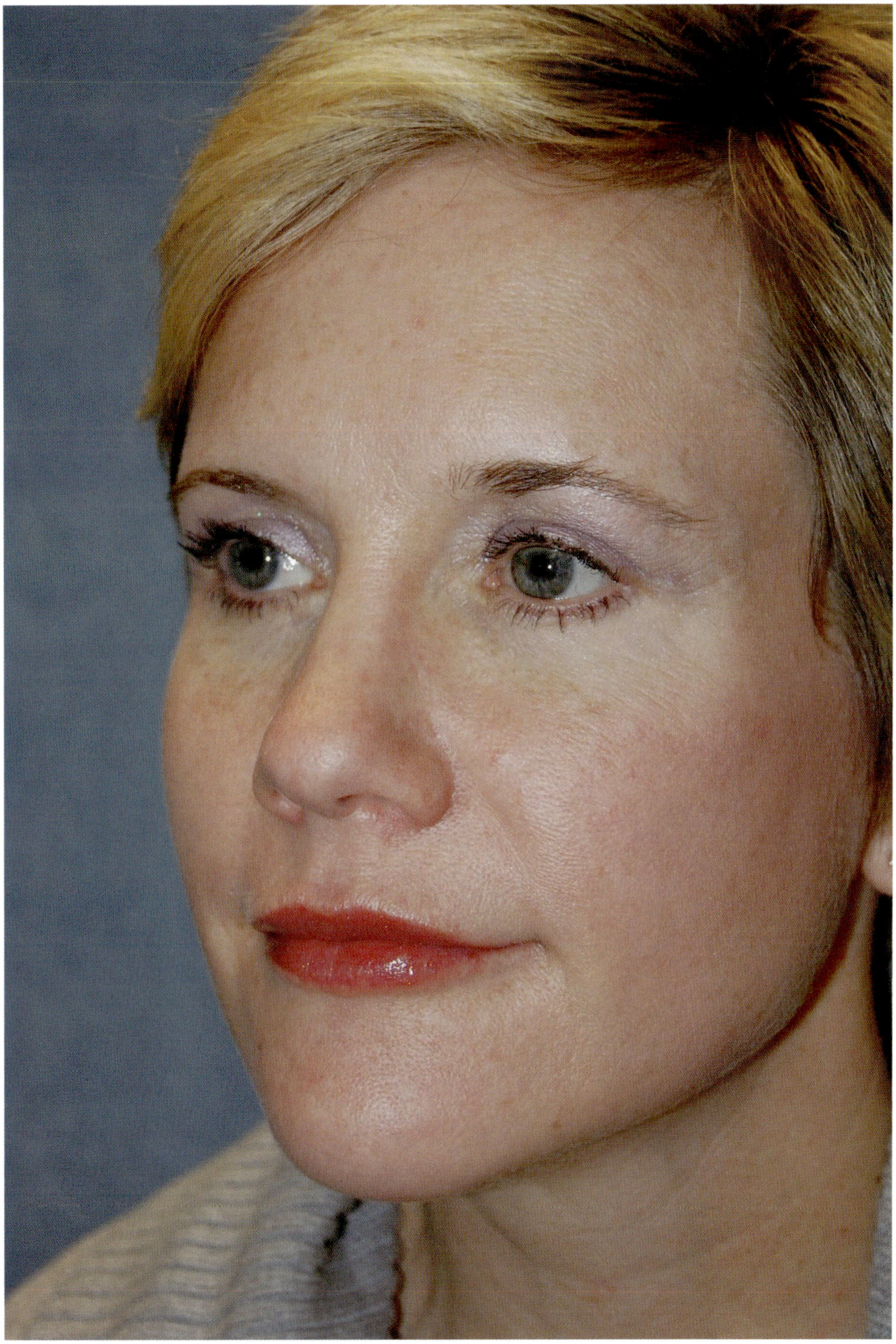

# Rhinoplasty Case 1

Front view

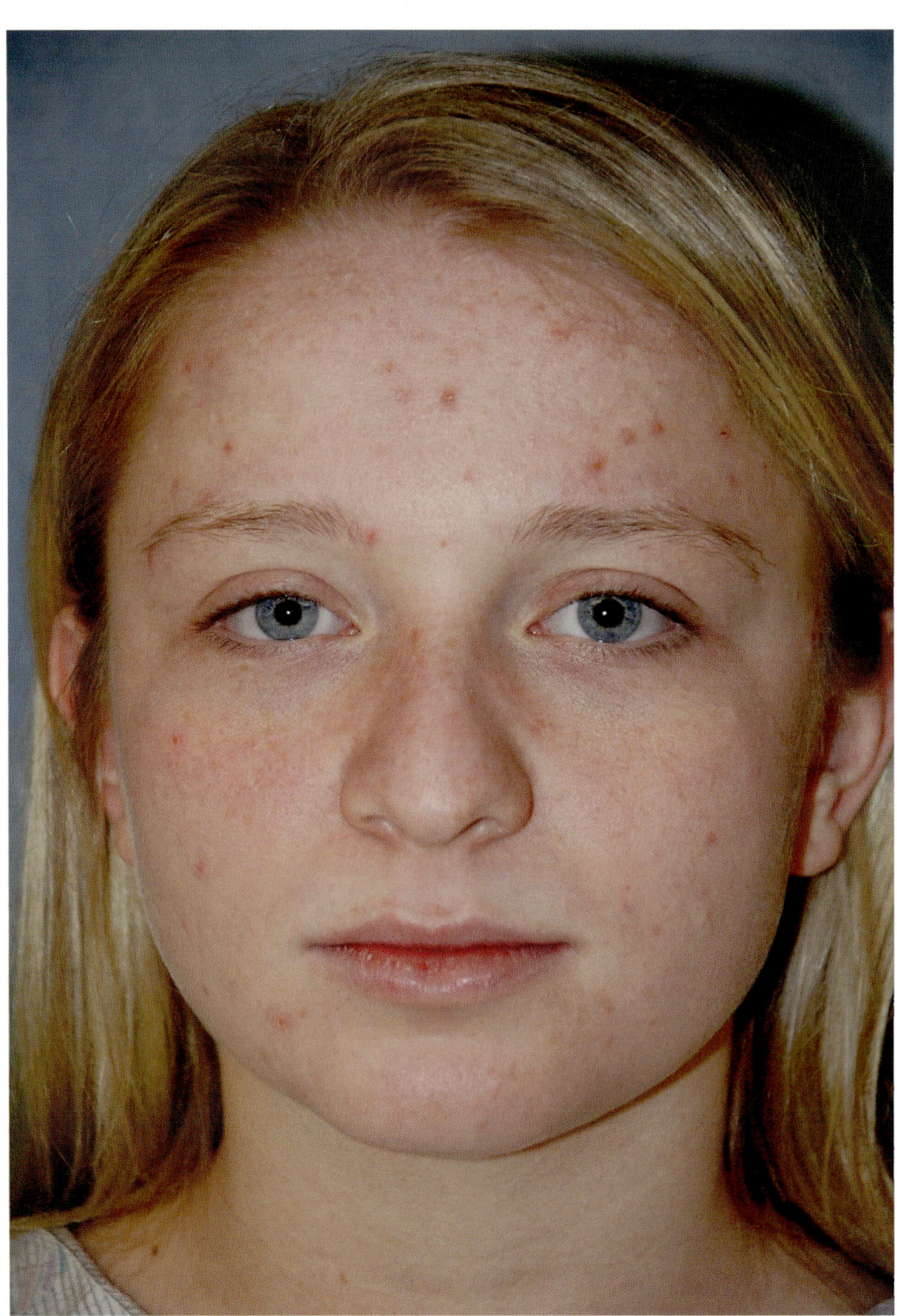

Front view

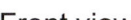

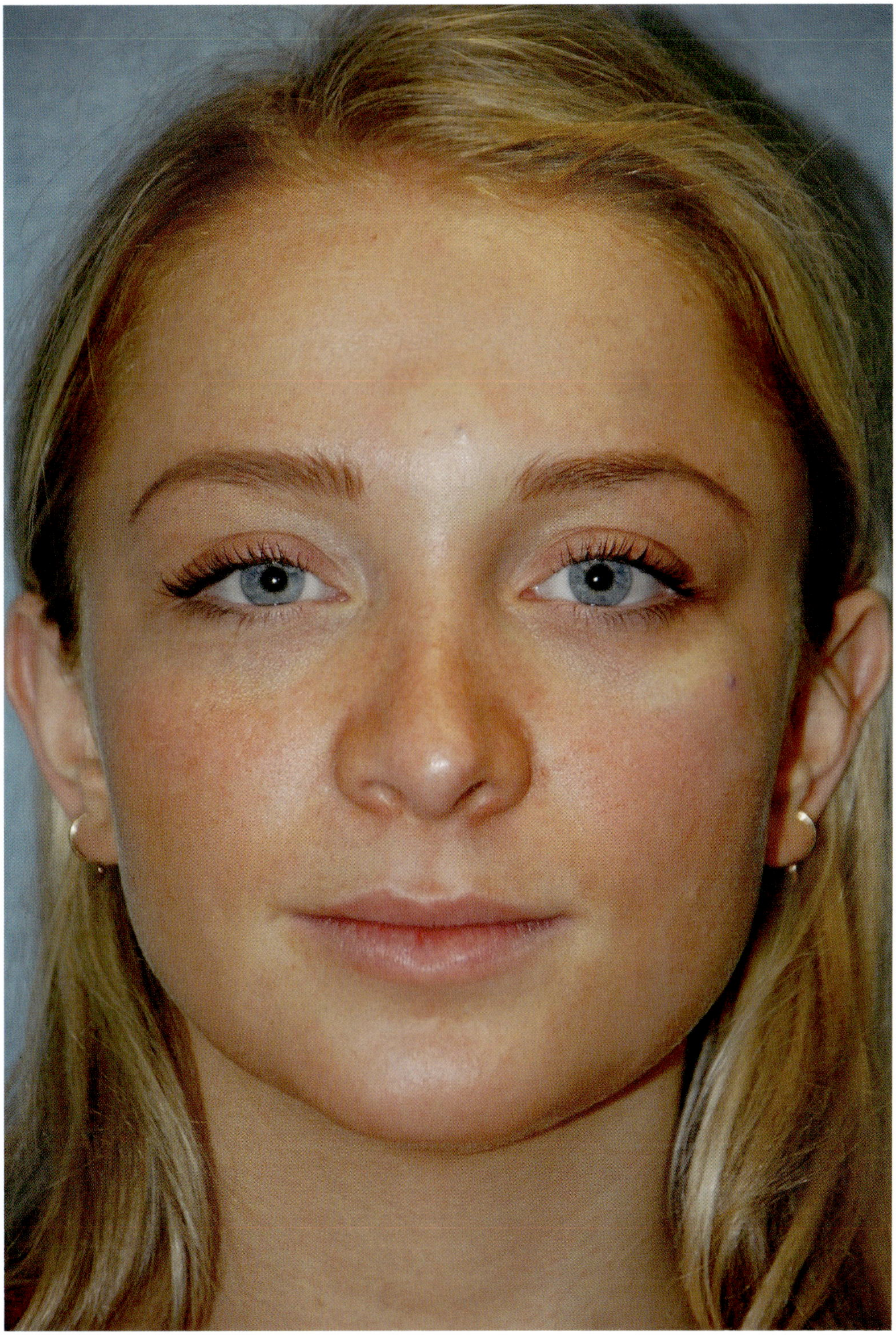

Angle view

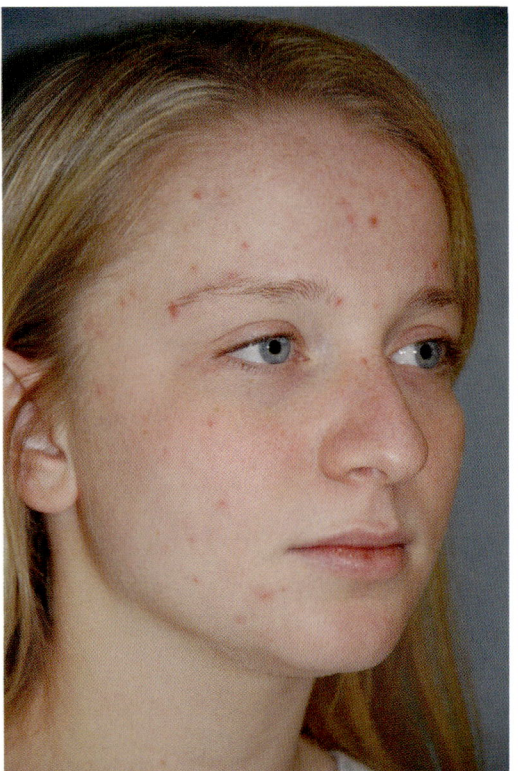
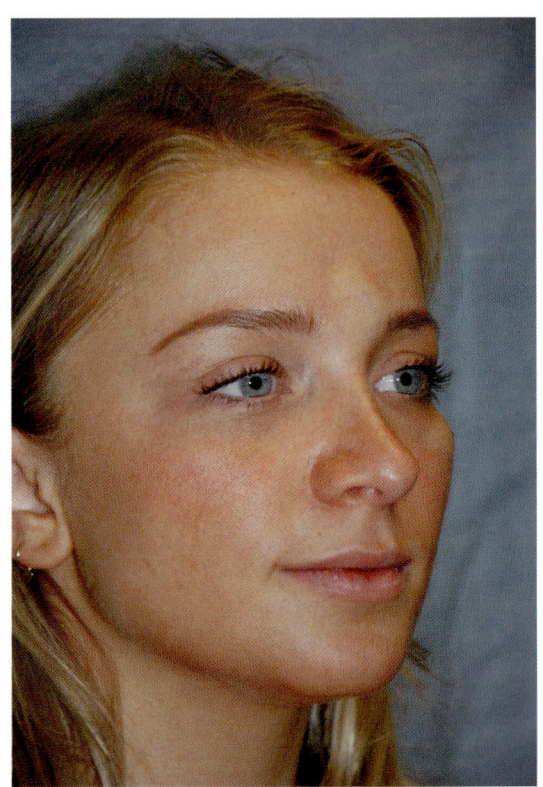

Side view

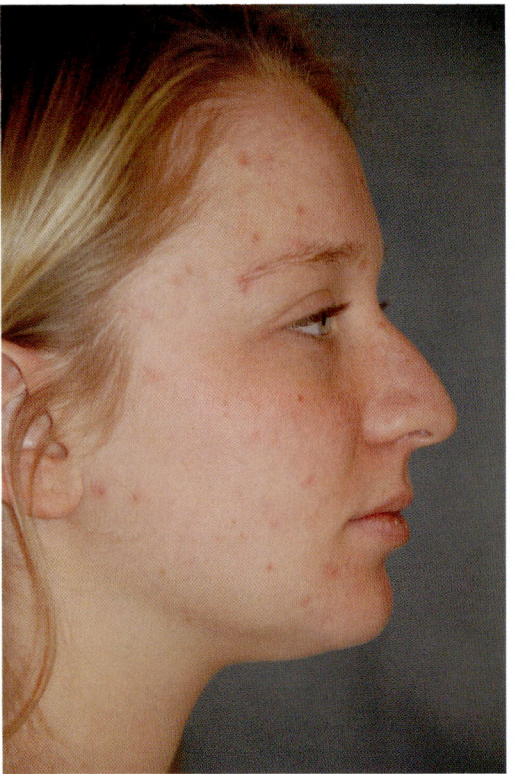
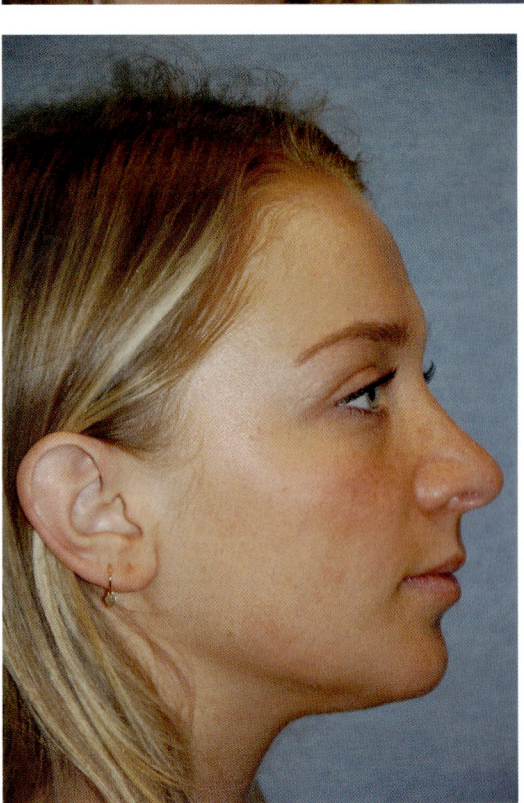

# Rhinoplasty Case 2

Front view

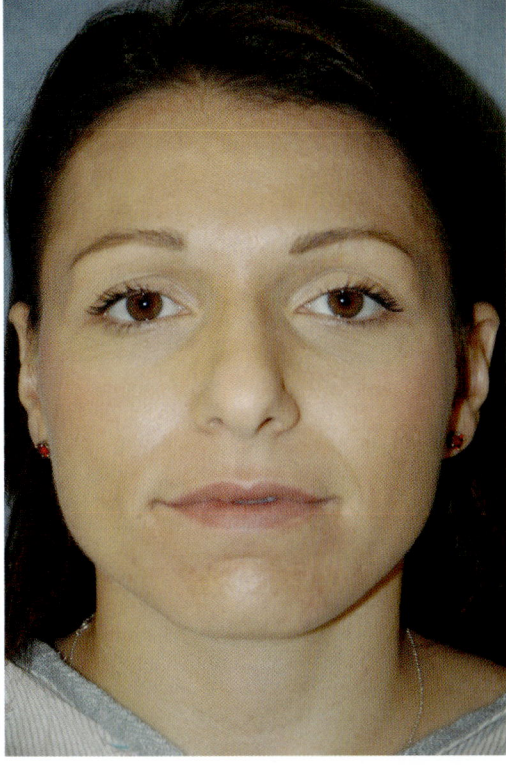 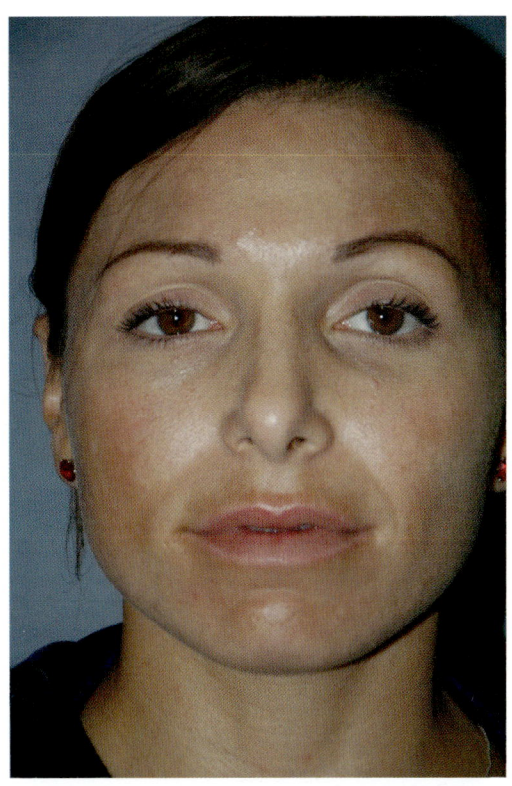

Angle view

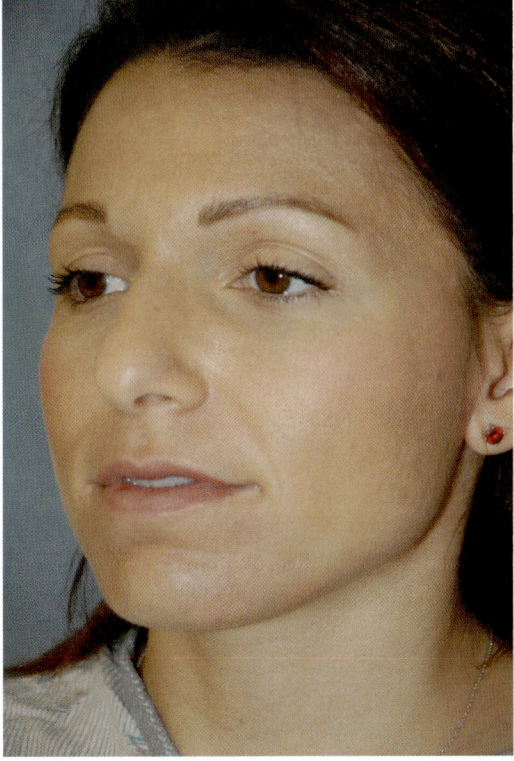 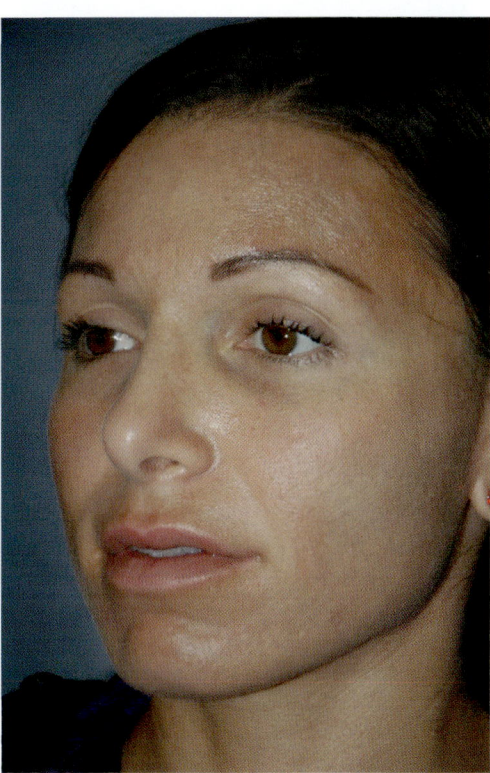

Side view

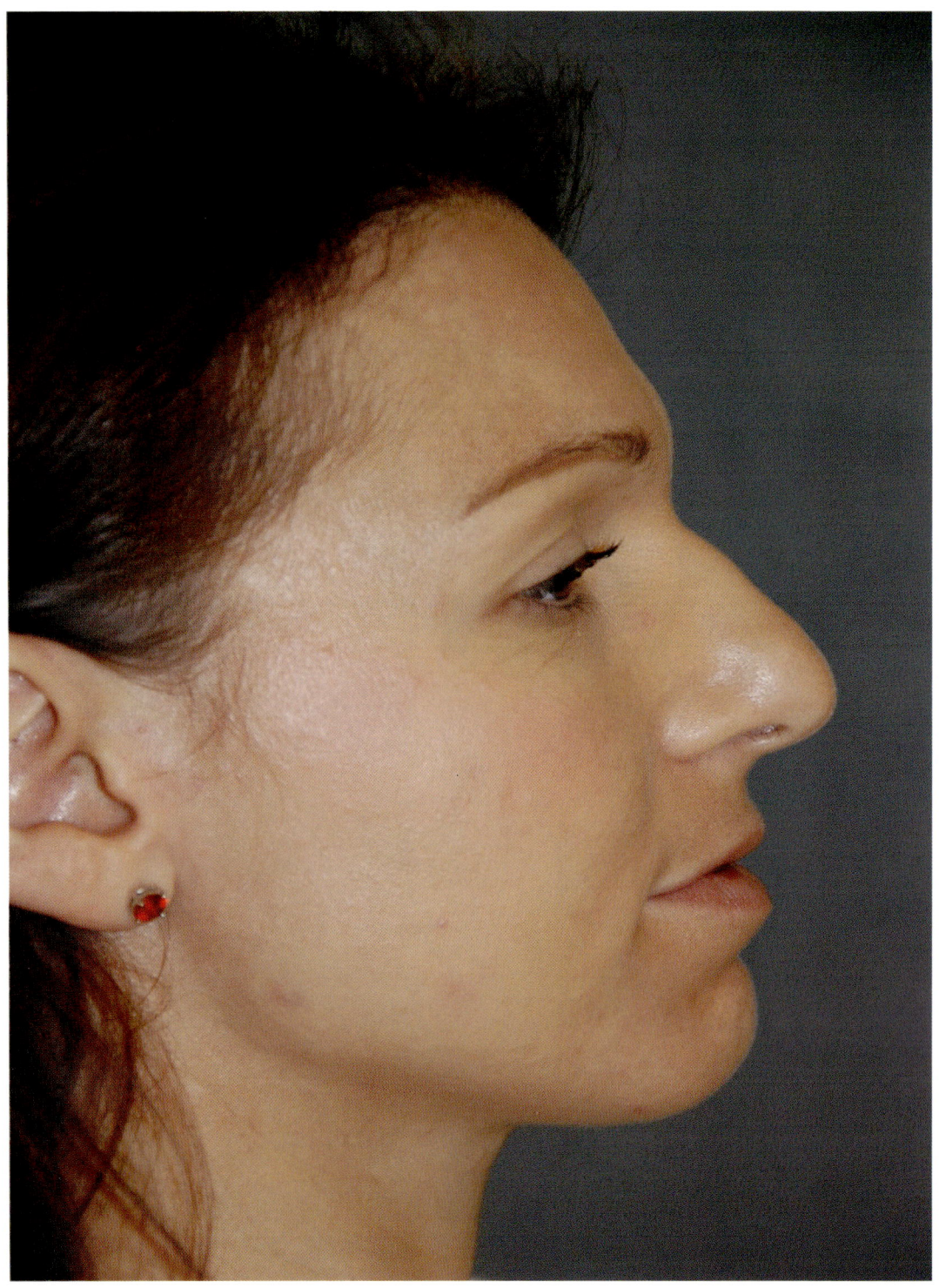

Side view

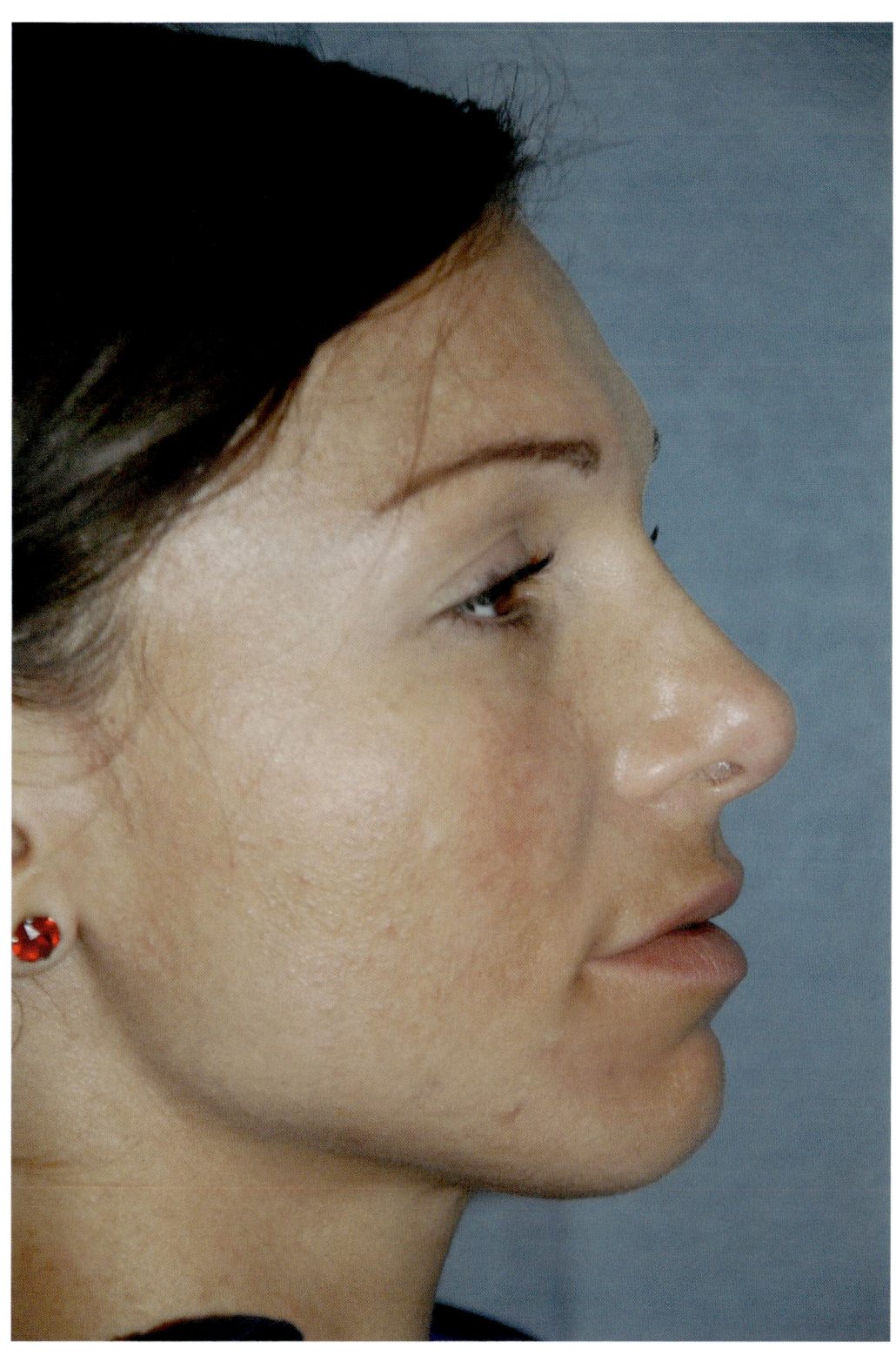

# Rhinoplasty Case 3

Front view

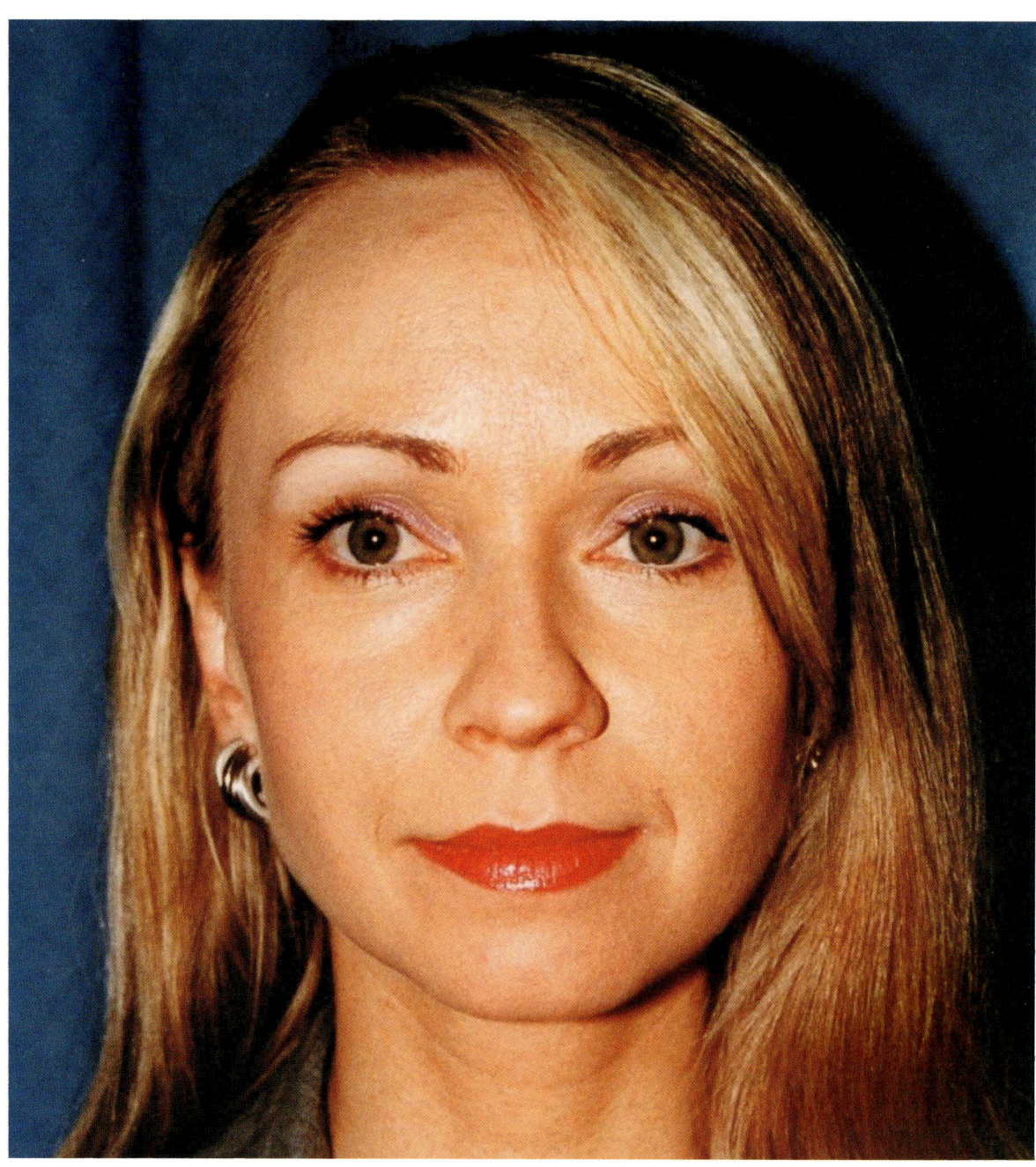

Front view

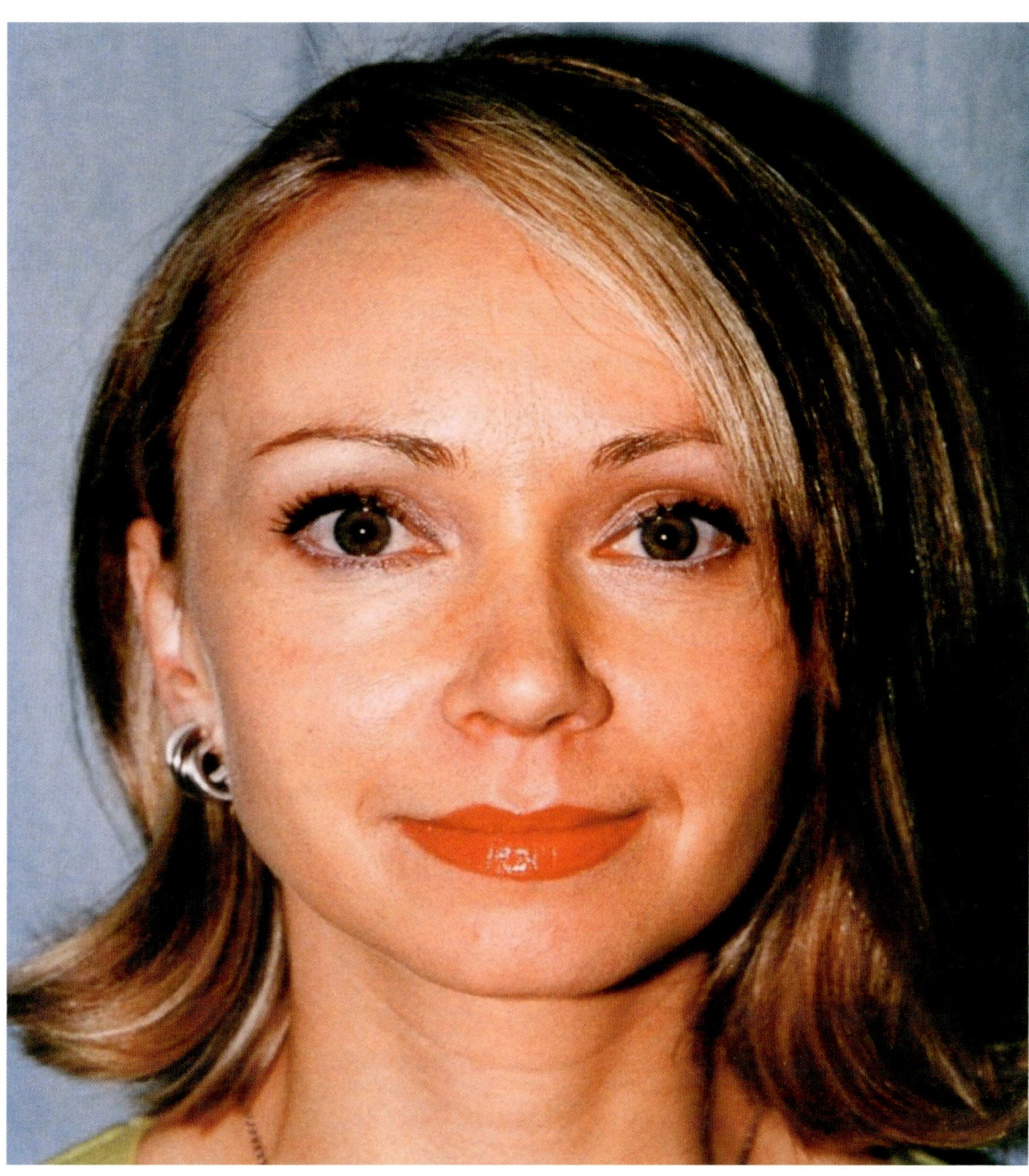

Angle and side view

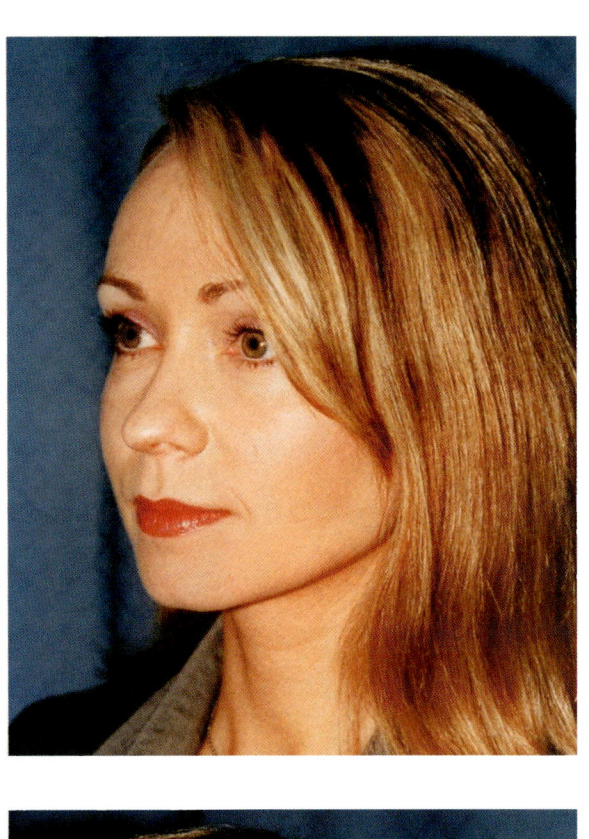
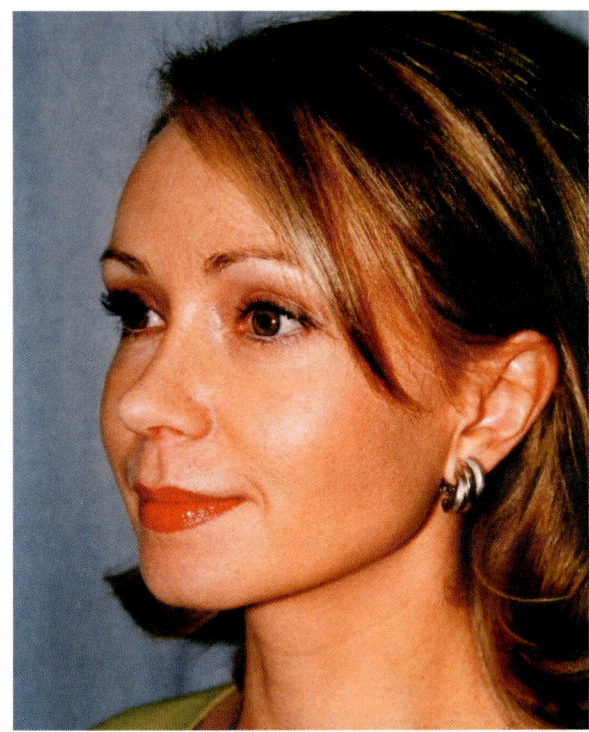
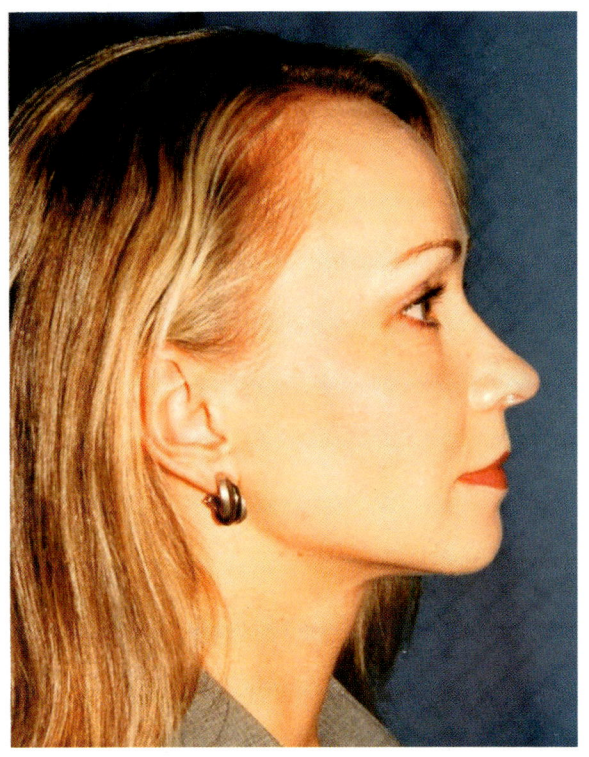
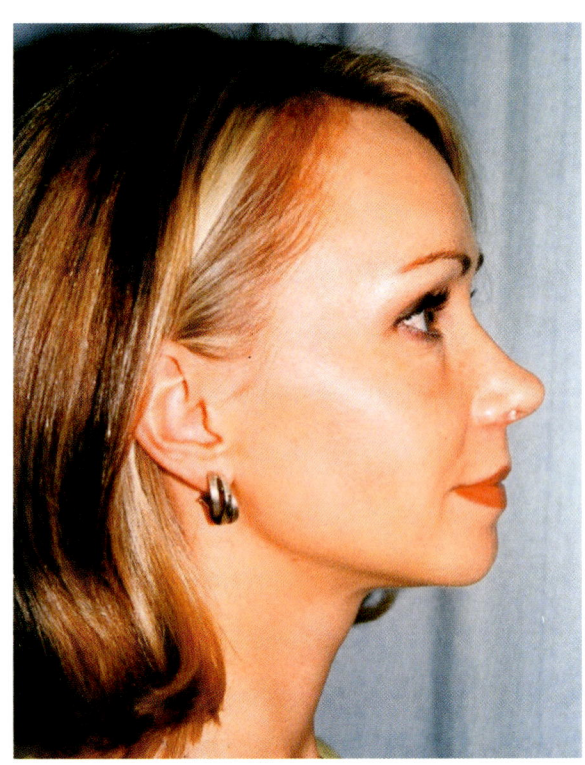

# Liposuction Case 1

Side and angle view

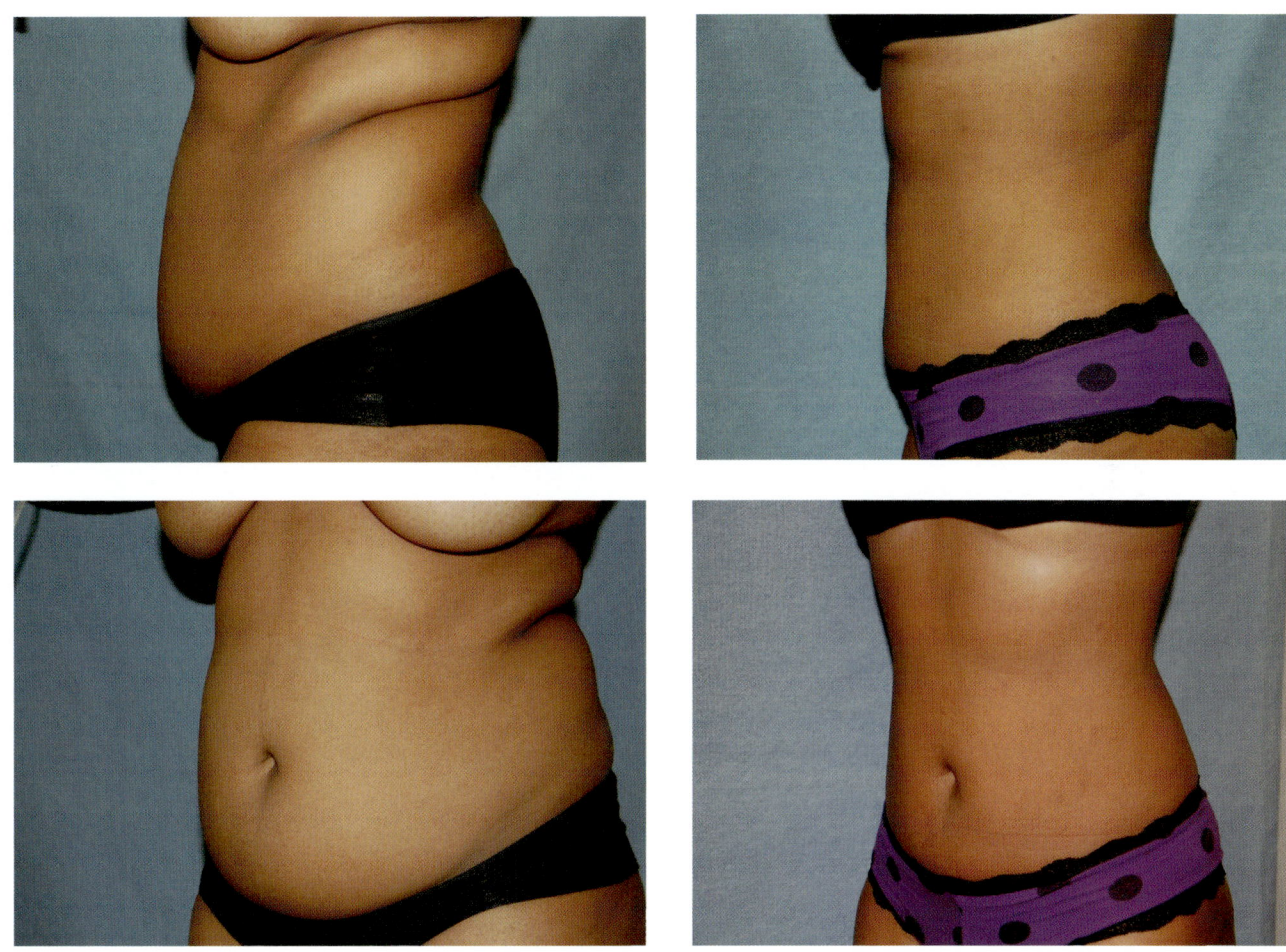

Front view

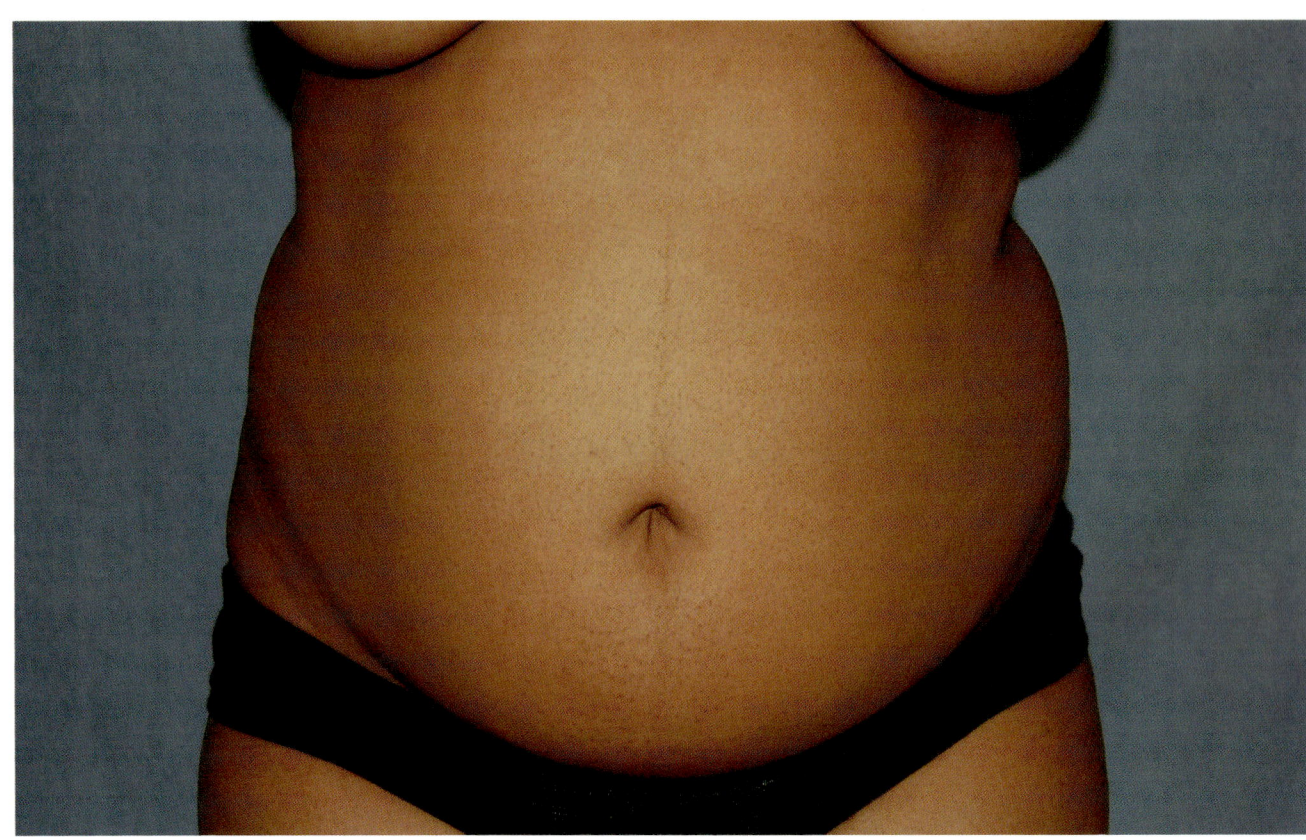

Front view

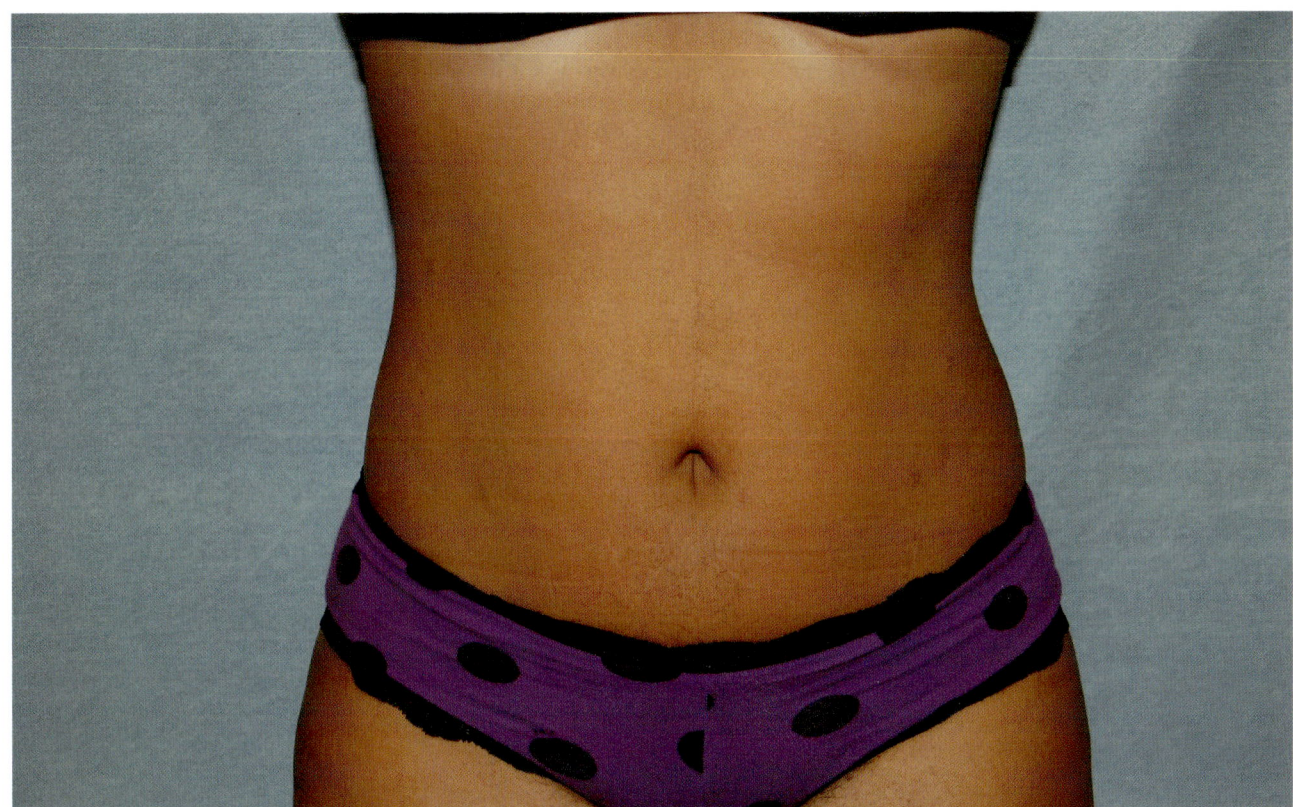

# Liposuction Case 2

Angle view

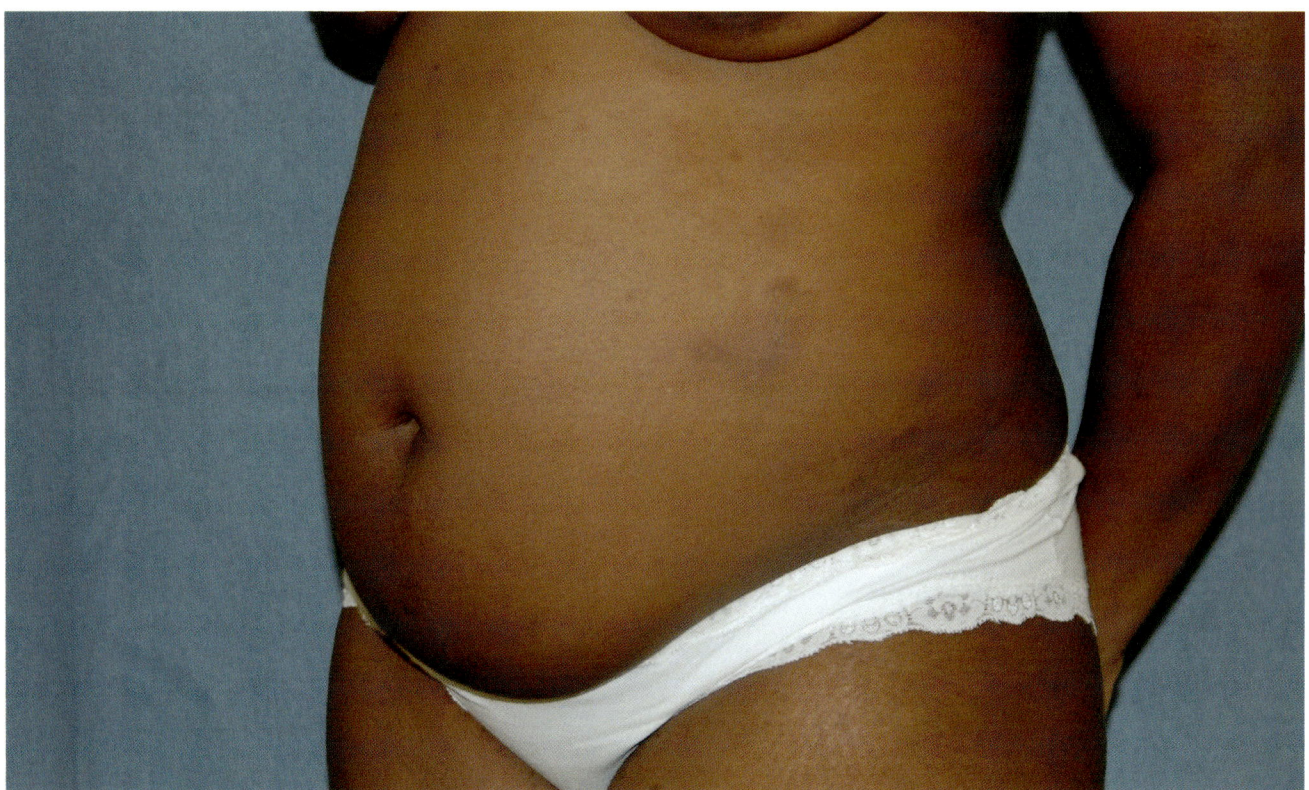

Angle view

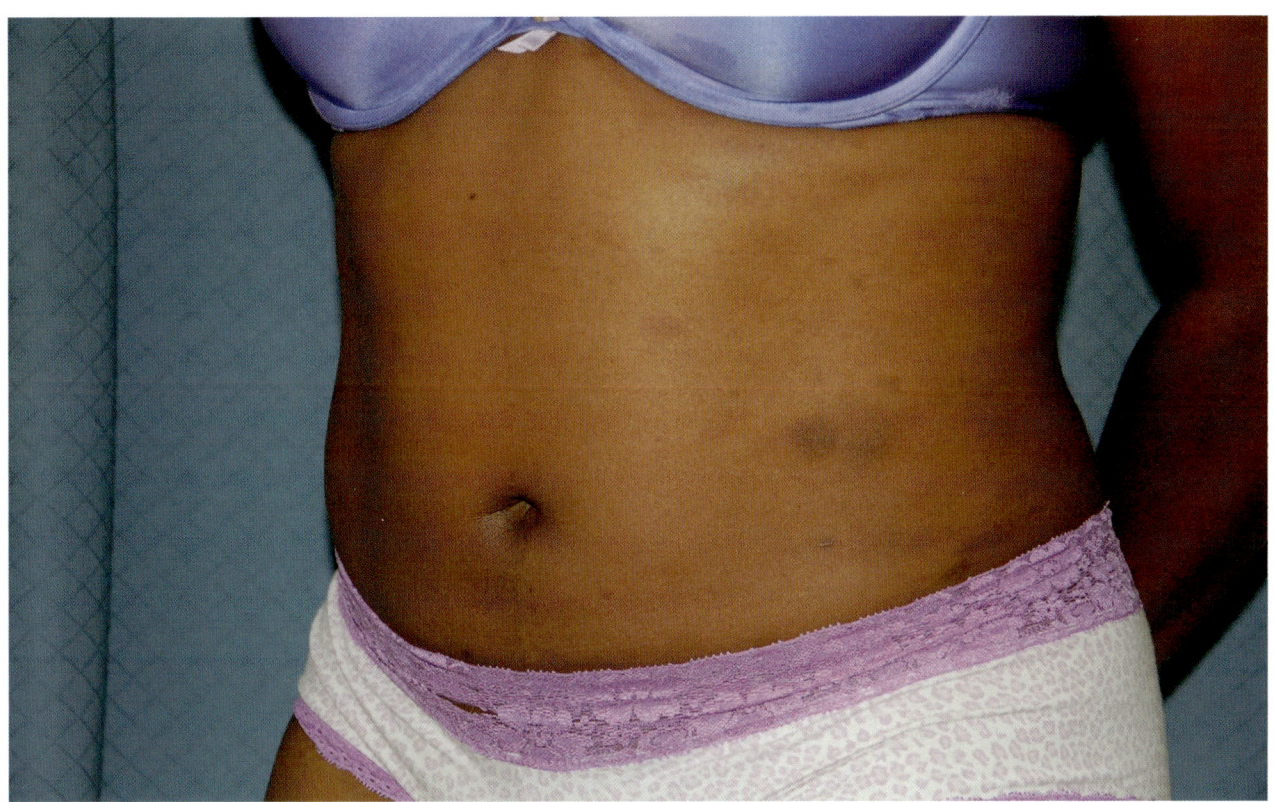

Front view

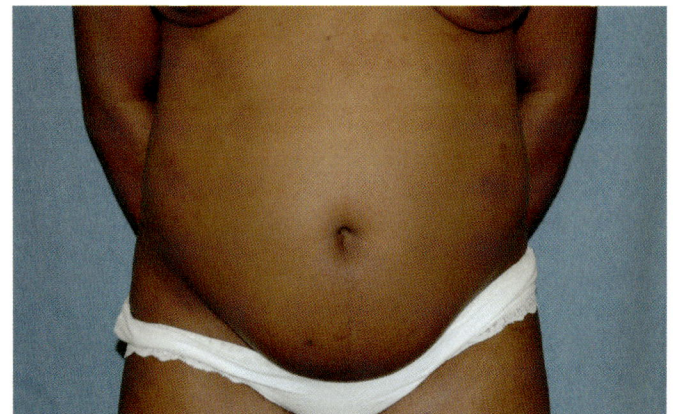 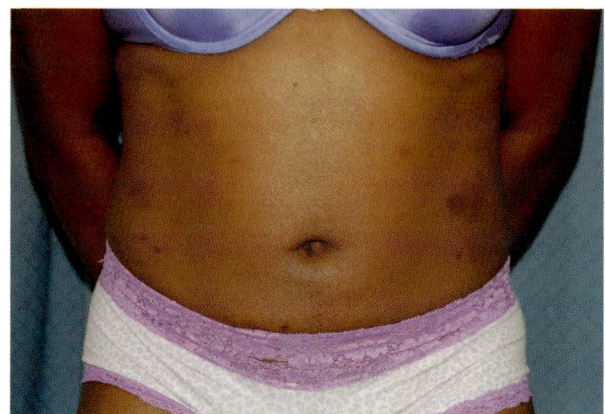

Side view

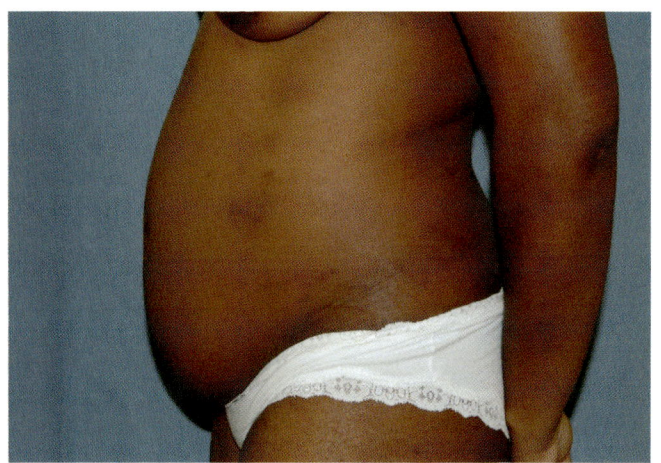 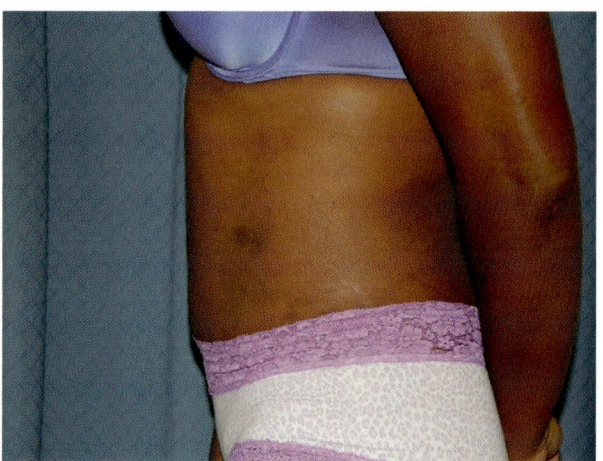

# Liposuction Case 3

Front view

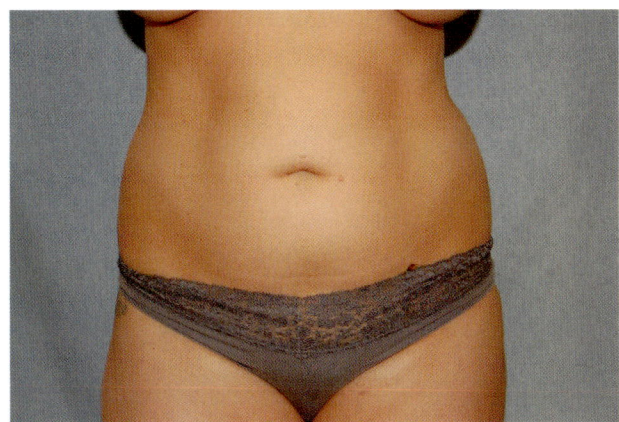 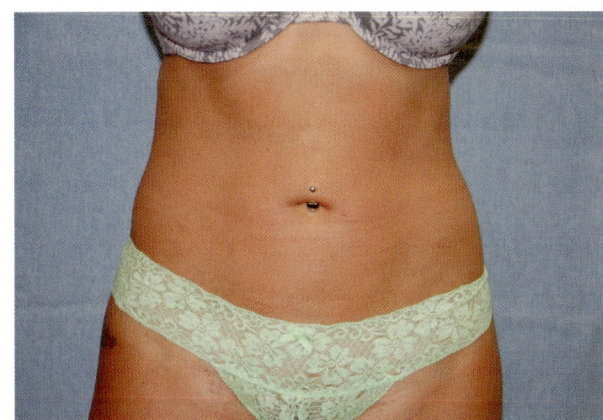

Angle view

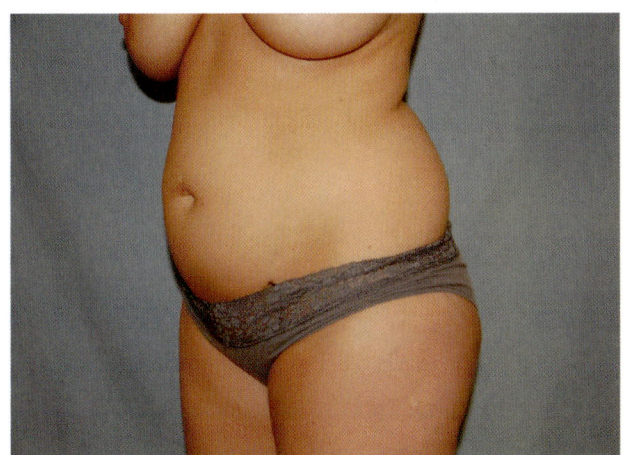 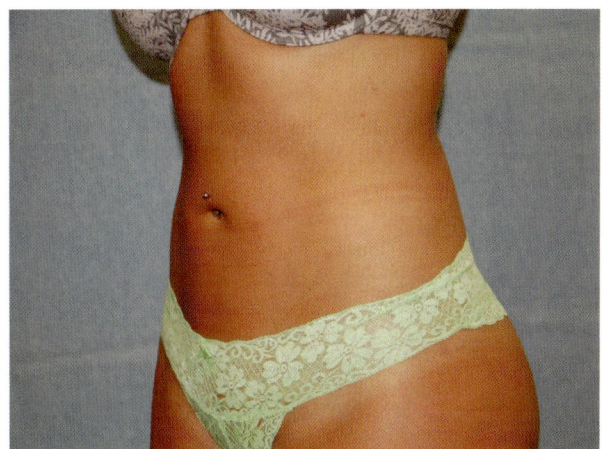

BBL Case 1

Angle view

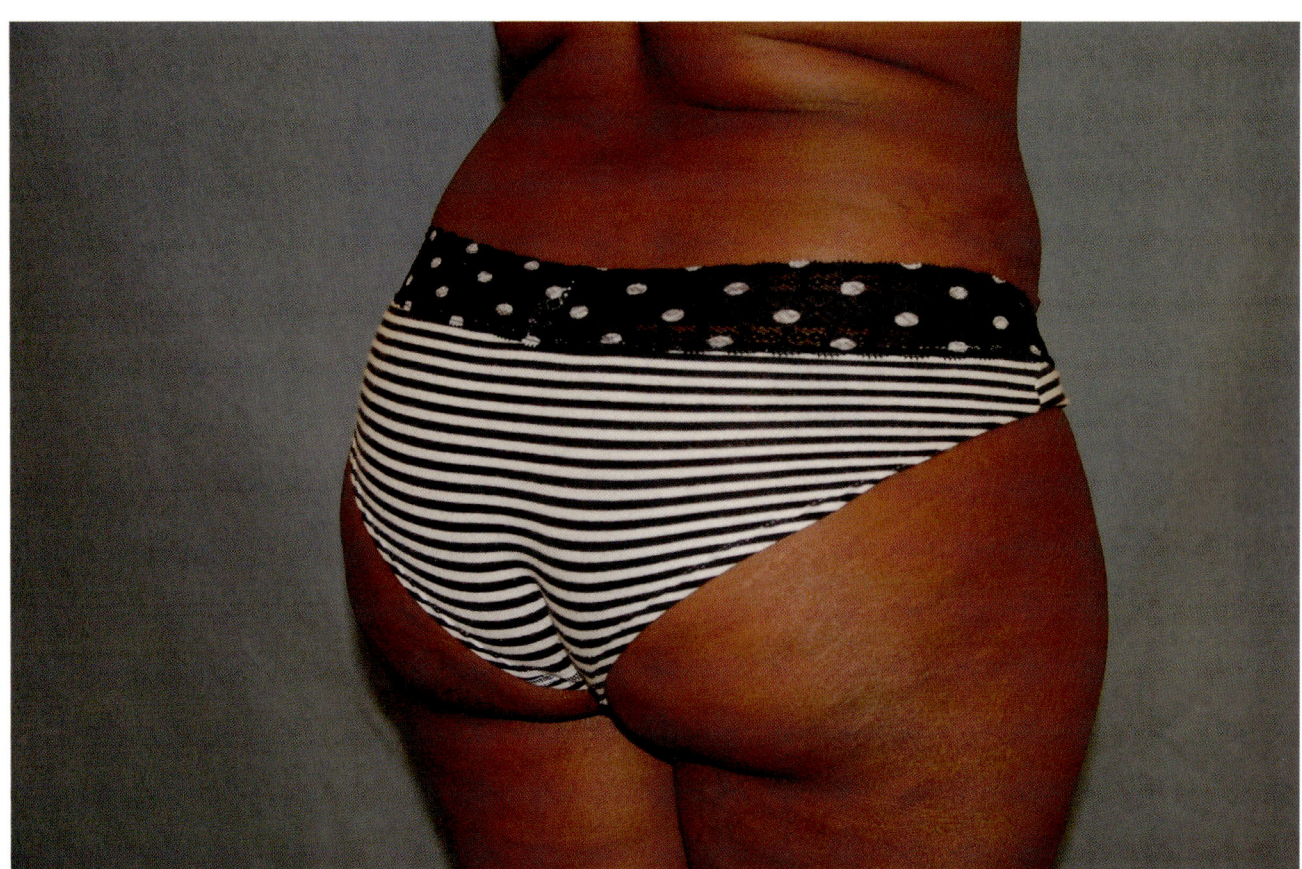

Angle view

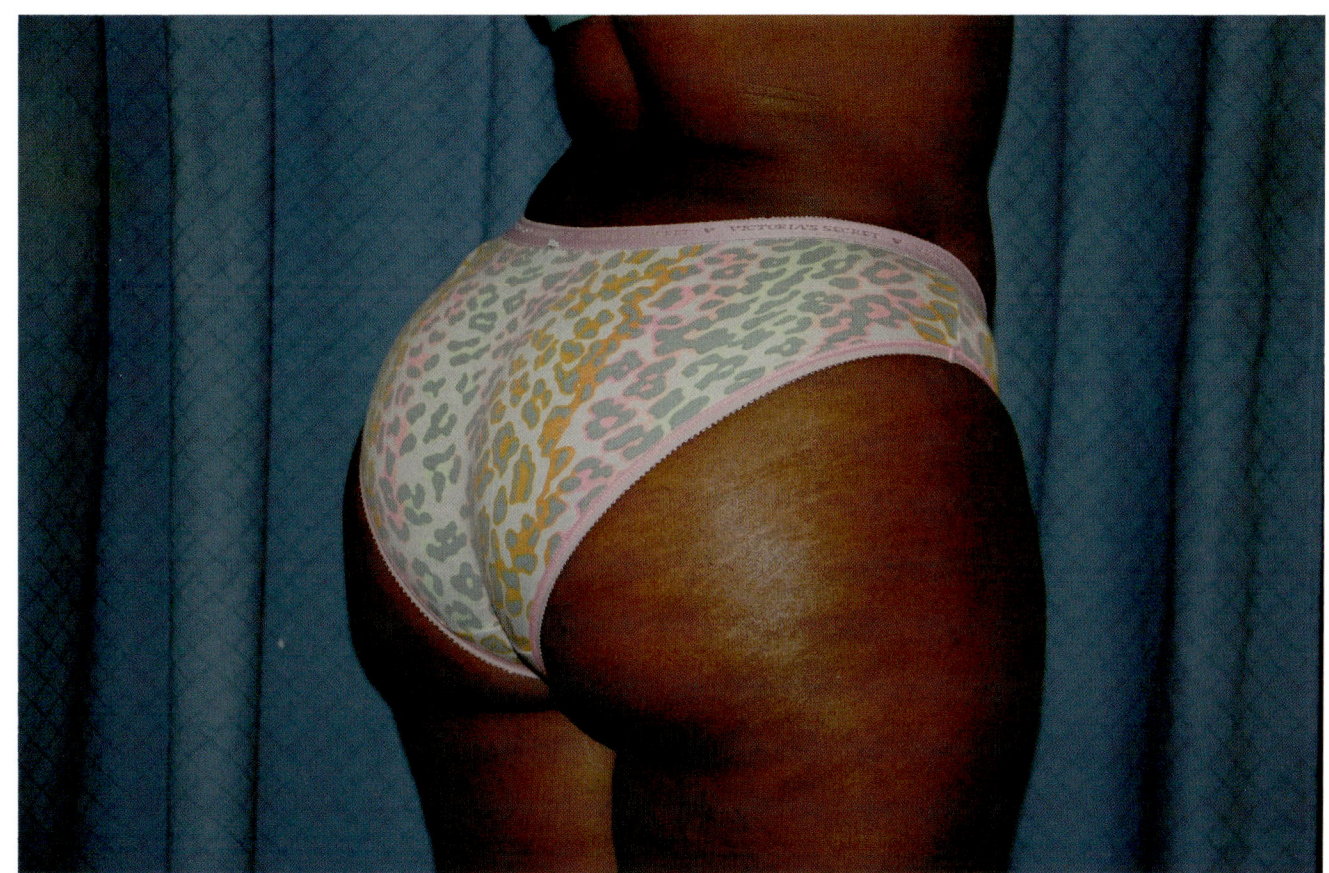

Front and angle view

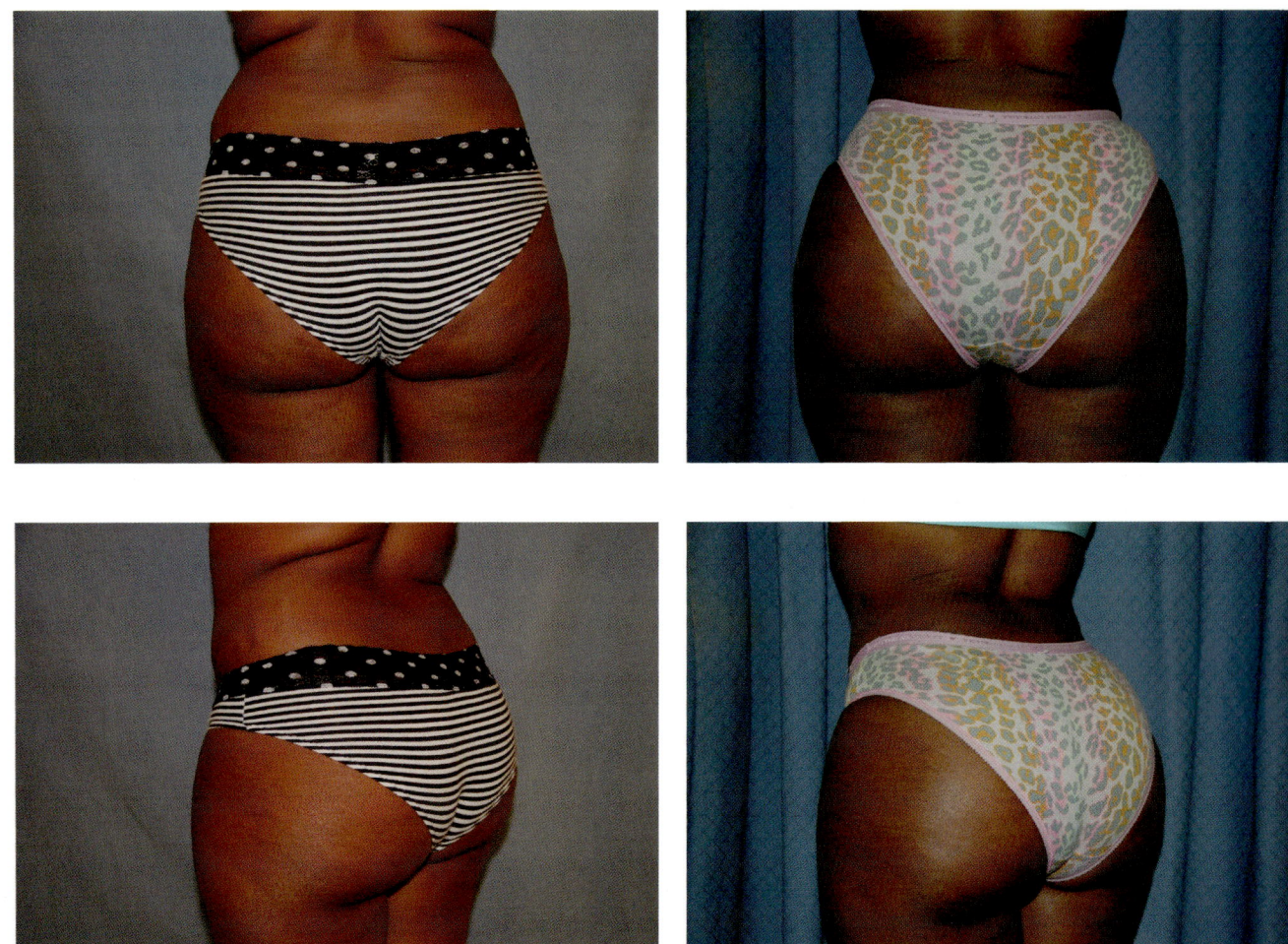

## BBL Case 2

Angle, front, and side view

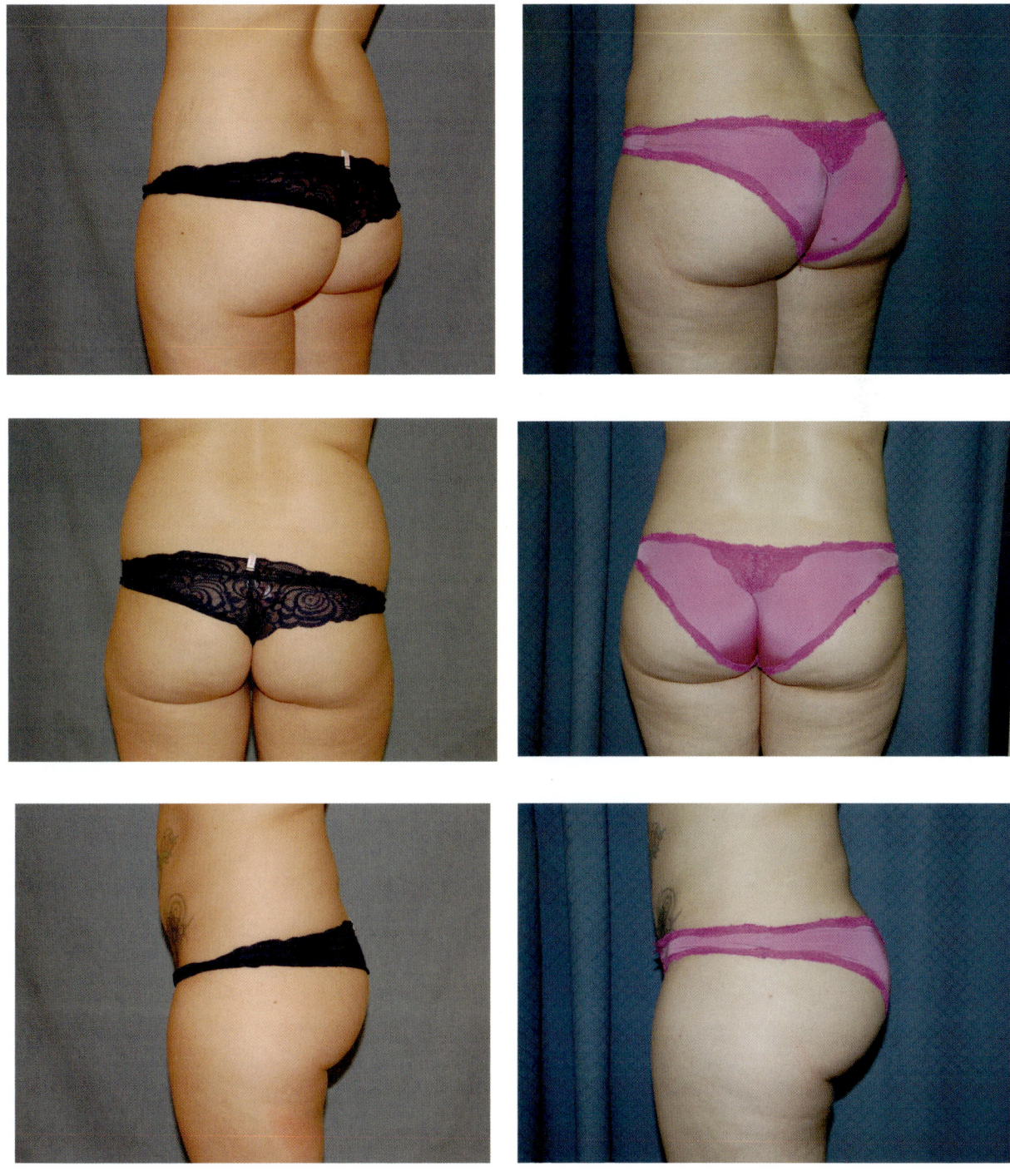

BBL Case 3

Angle view

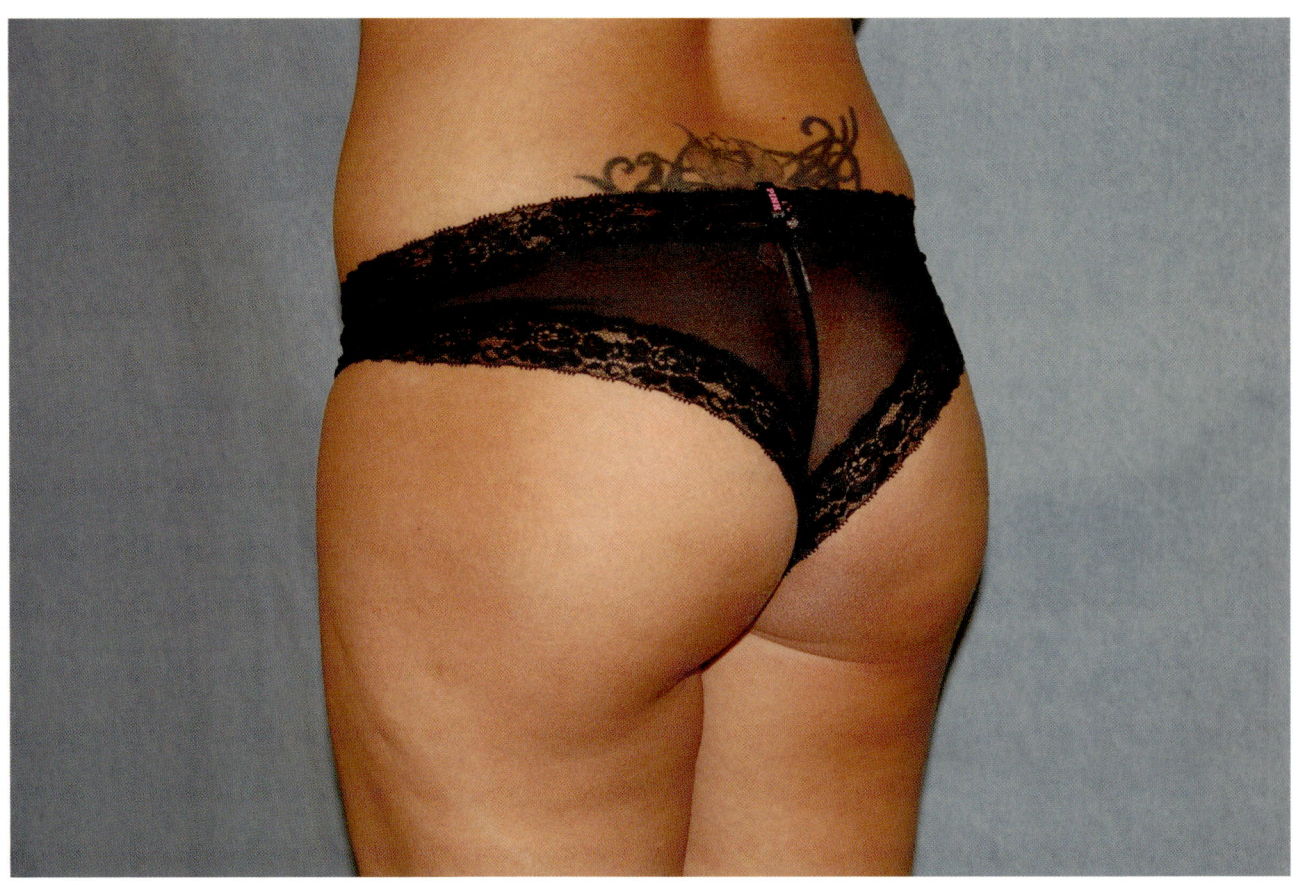

Angle view

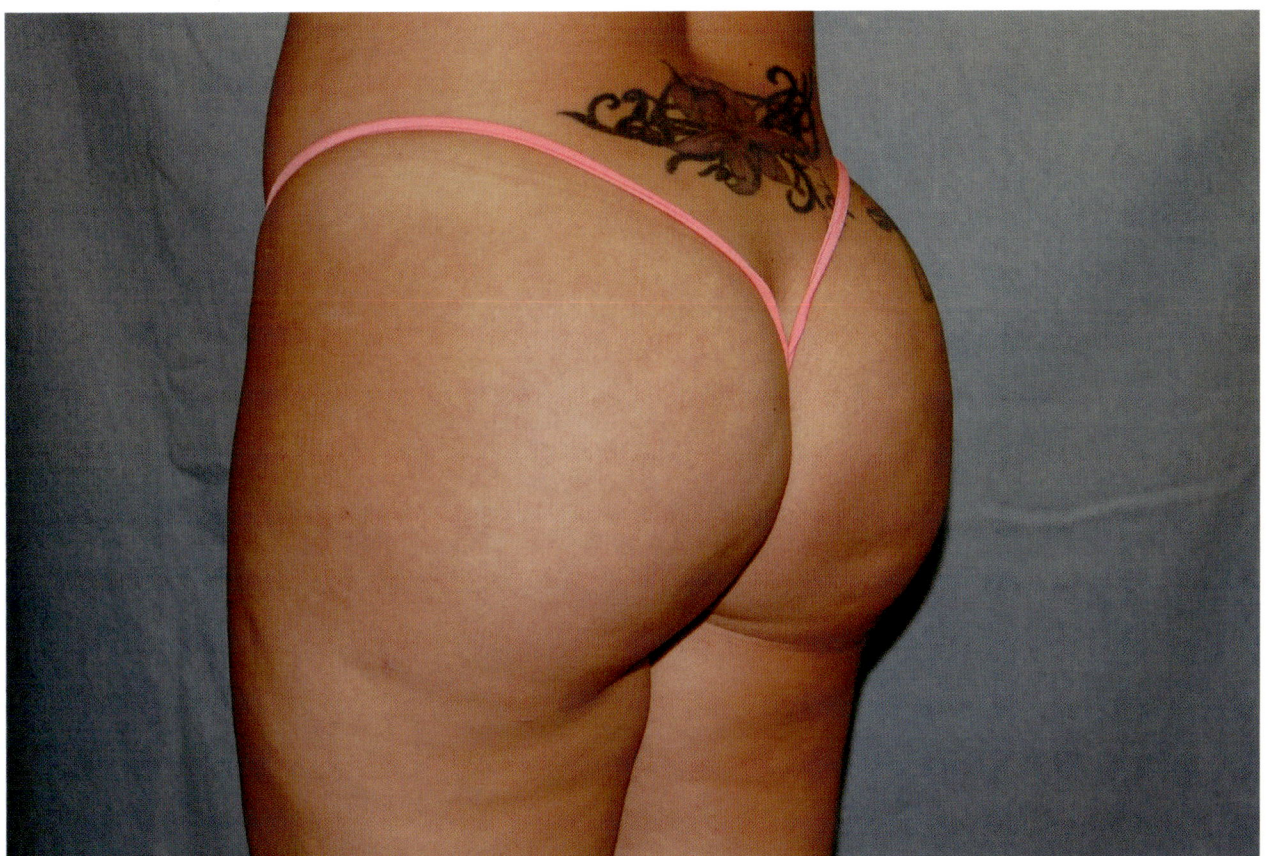

Side and front view

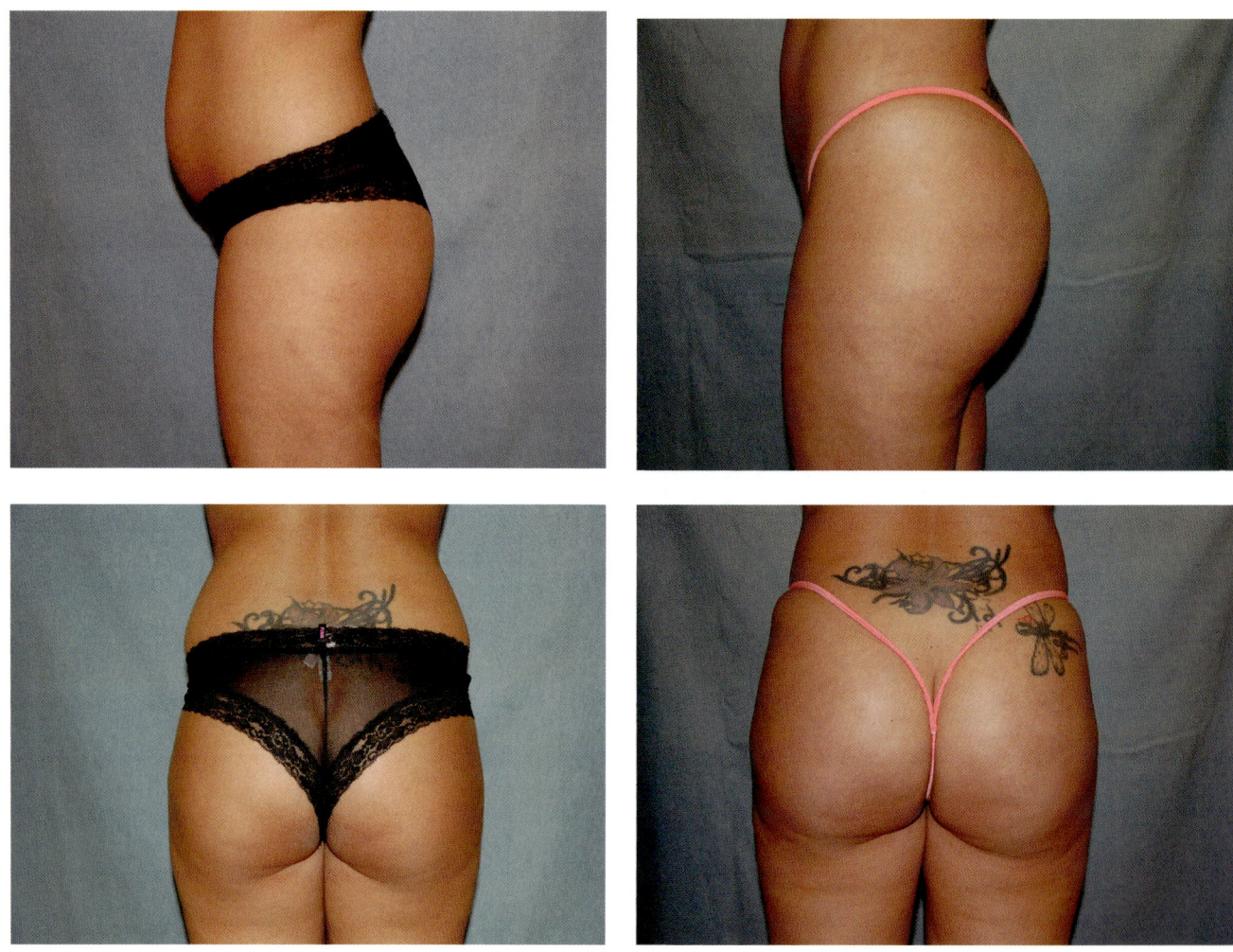

# Body, Thigh, Arm, and Butt Lift Case 1

Front, angle, and side view

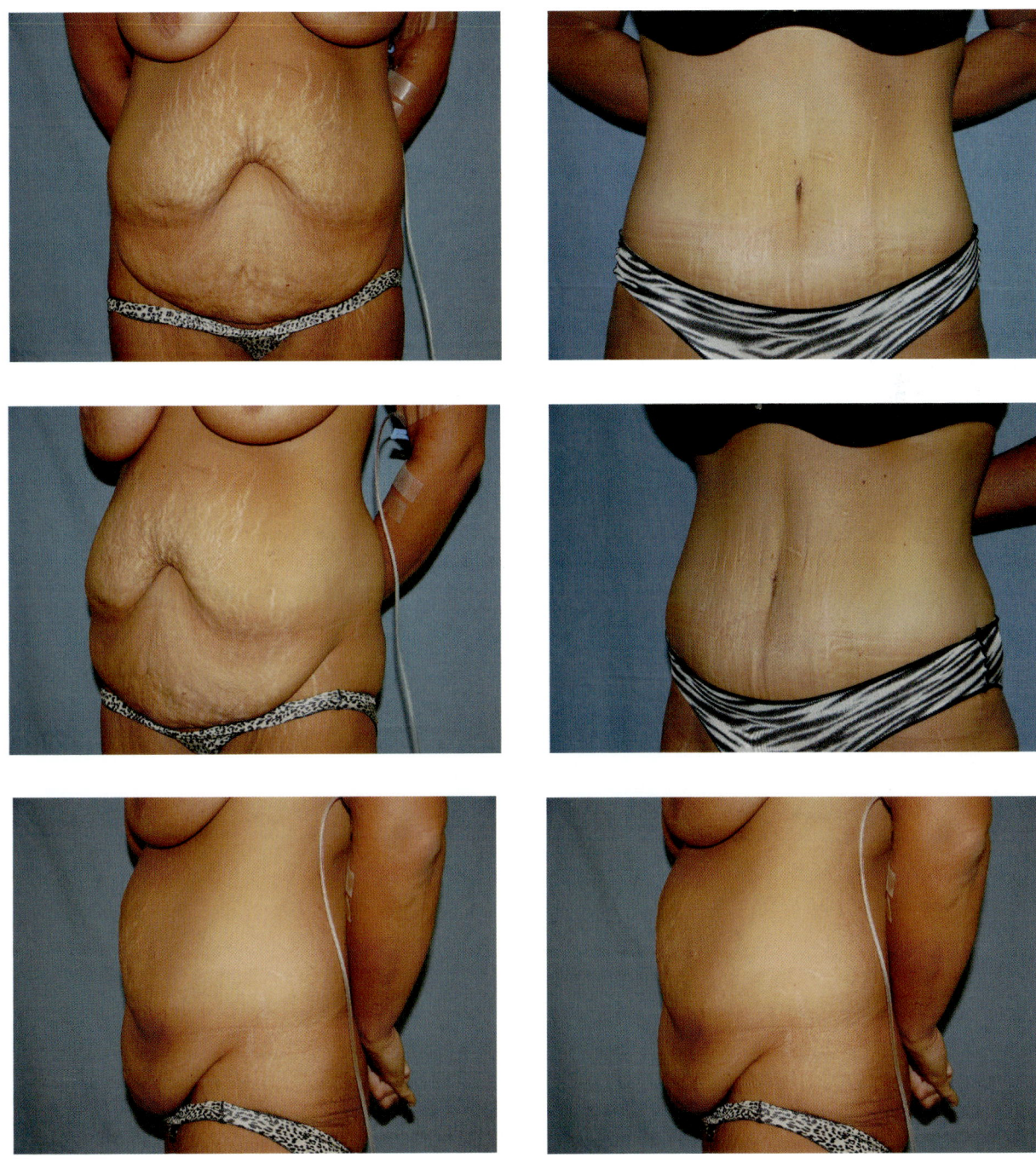

# Body, Thigh, Arm, and Butt Lift Case 2

Front view

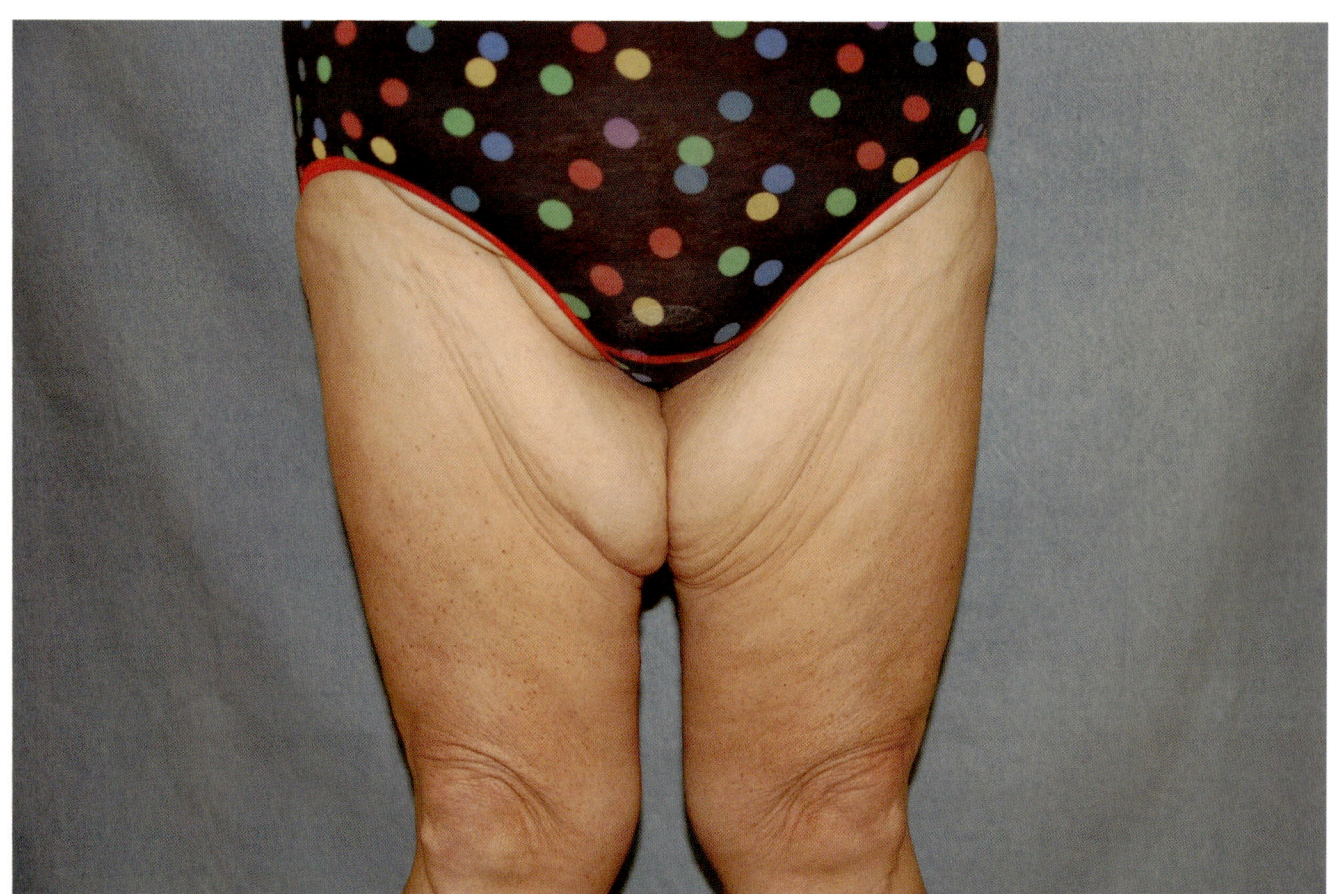

Front view

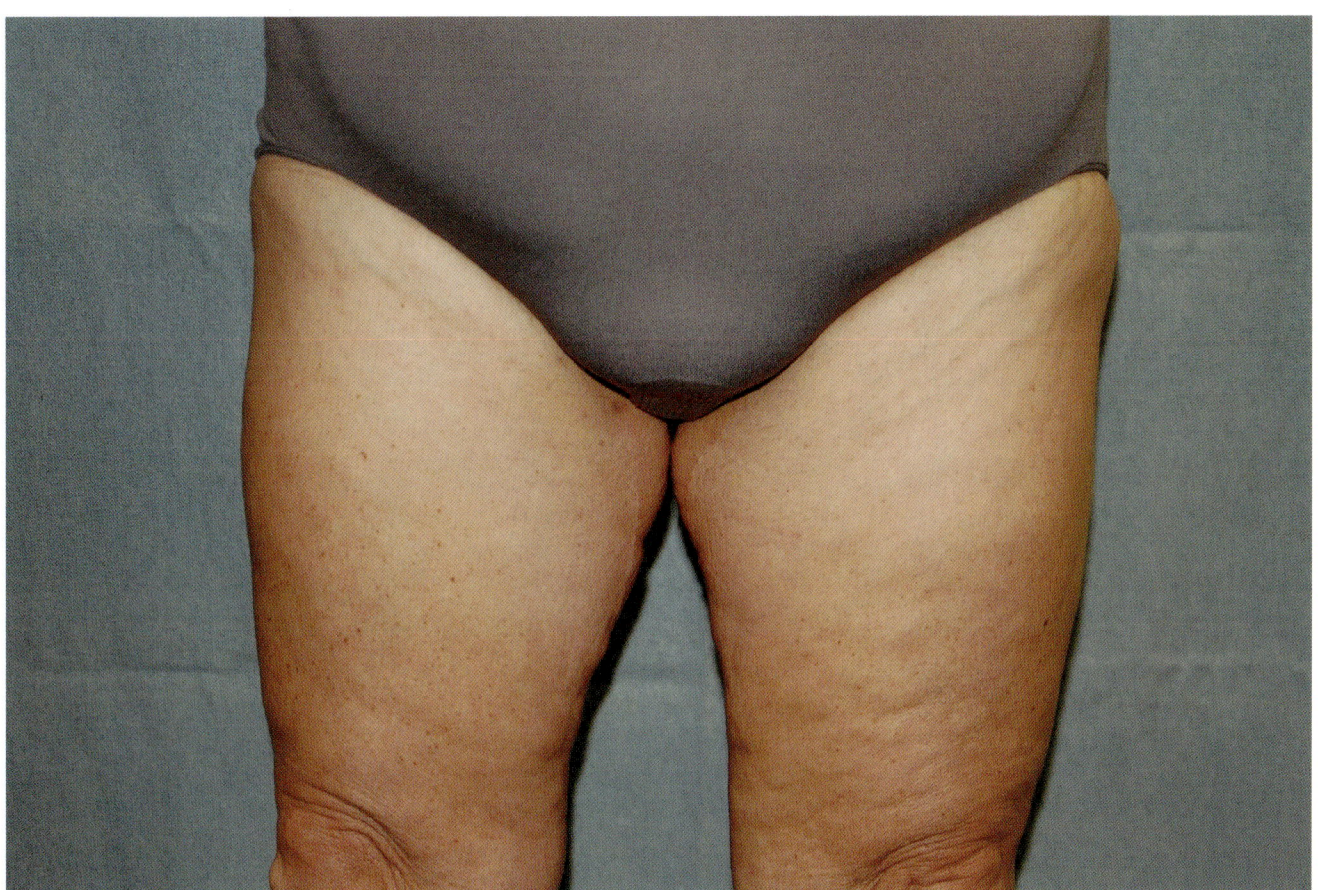

Angle and side view

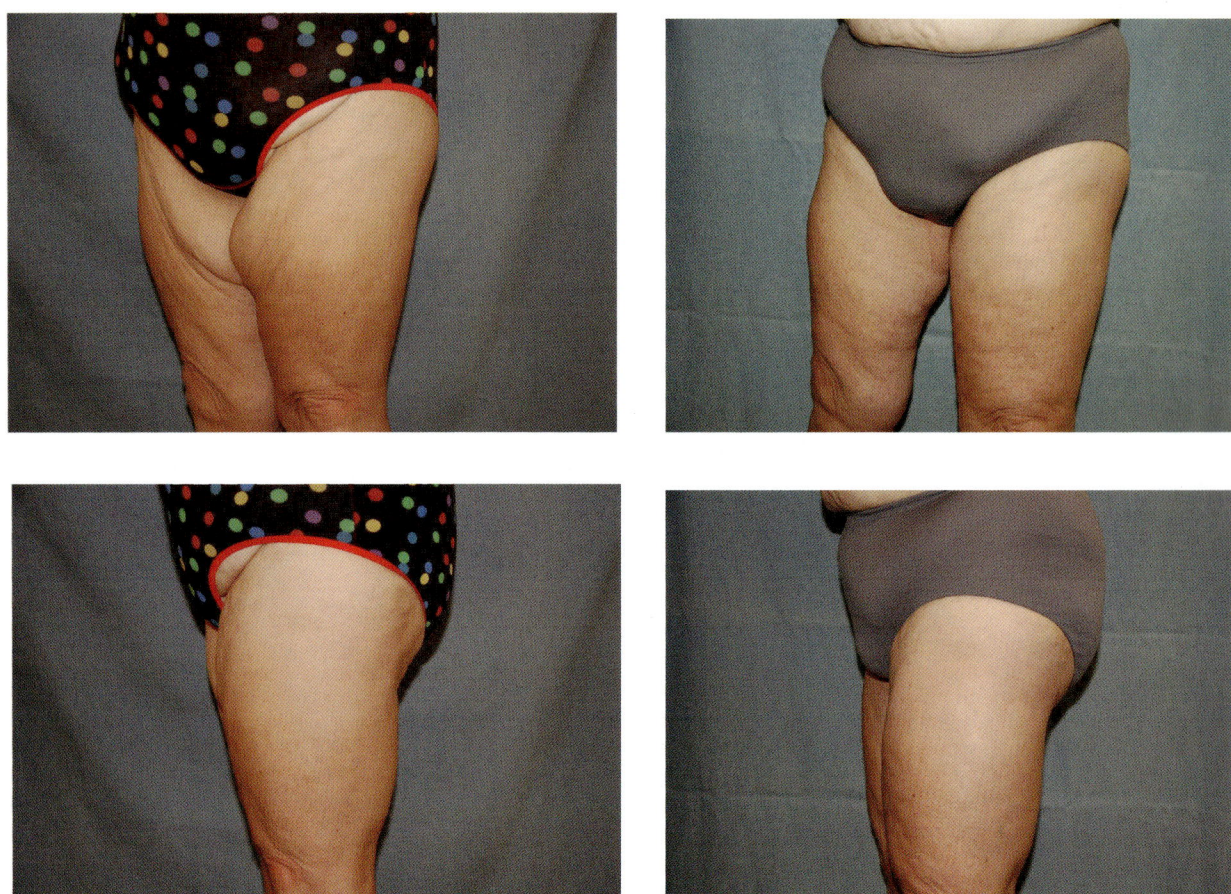

# Body, Thigh, Arm, and Butt Lift Case 3

Front, angle, and side view

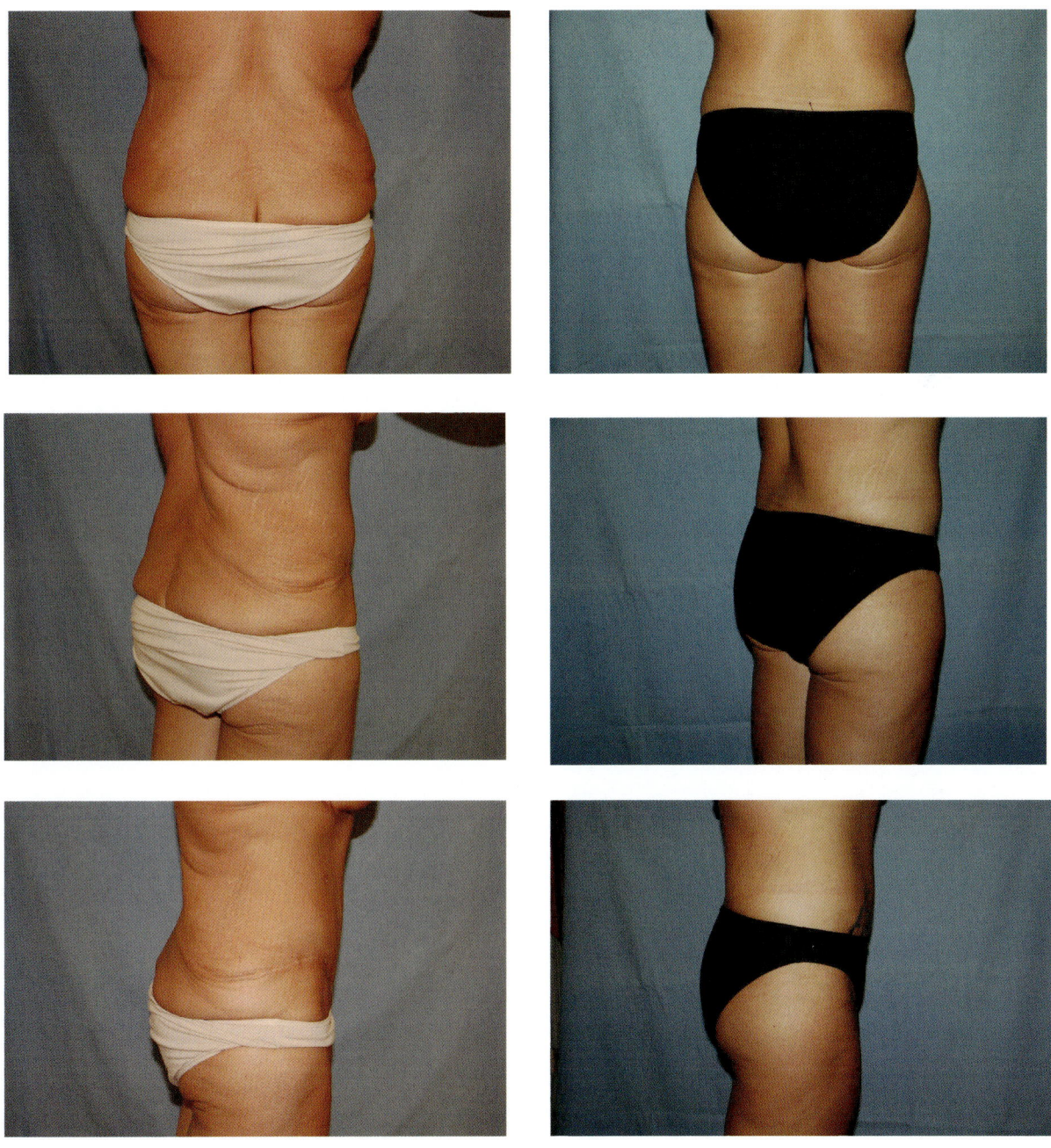

# Breast Lift and Reduction Case 1

Angle view

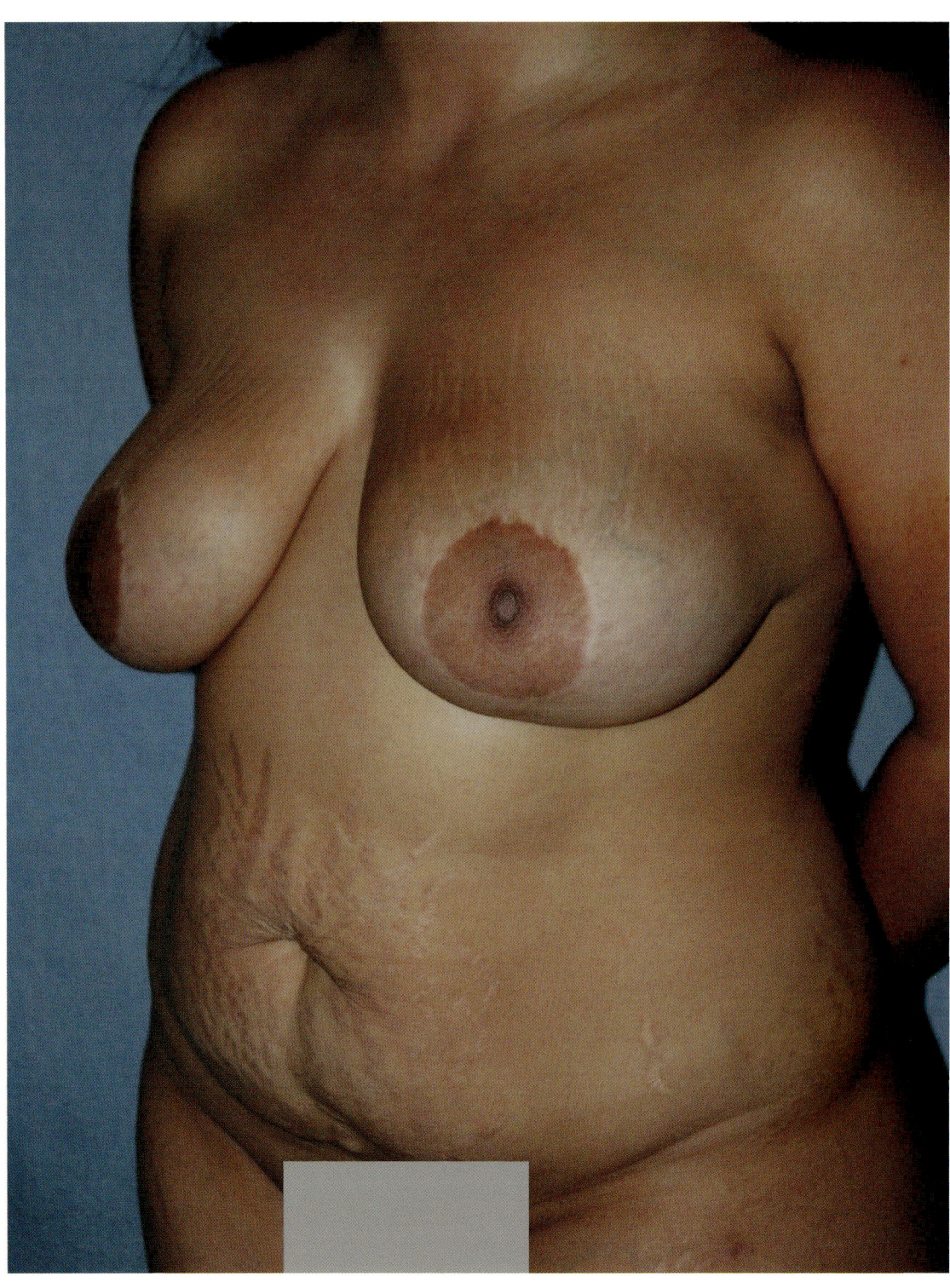

Angle view

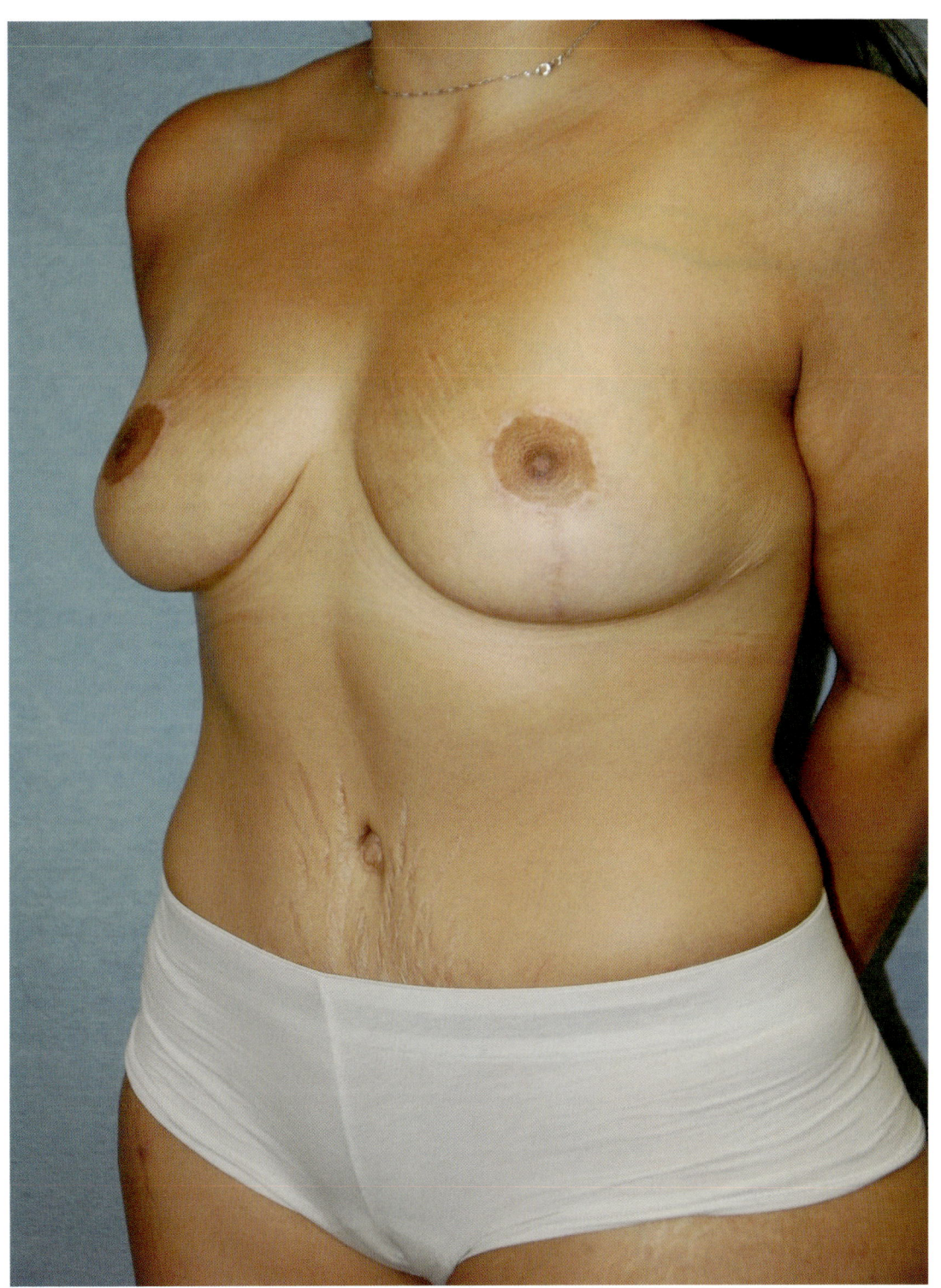

Front view

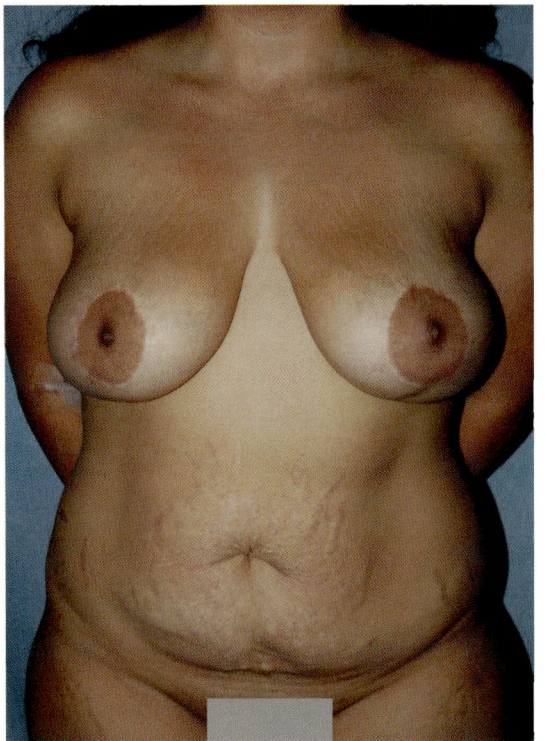 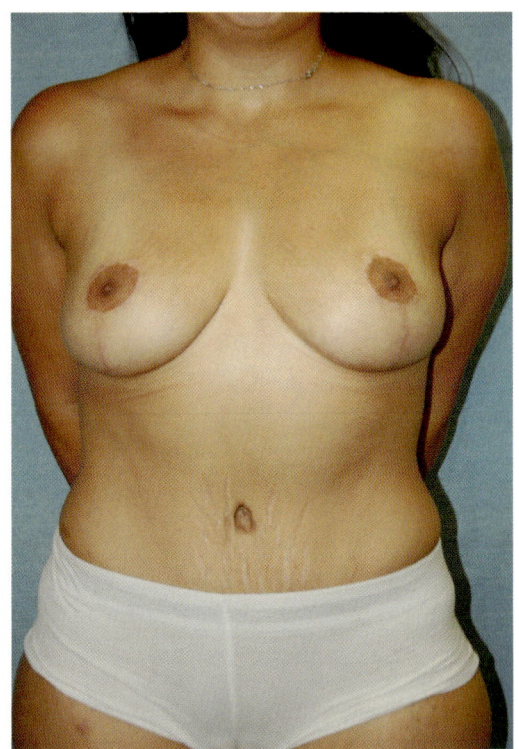

Side view

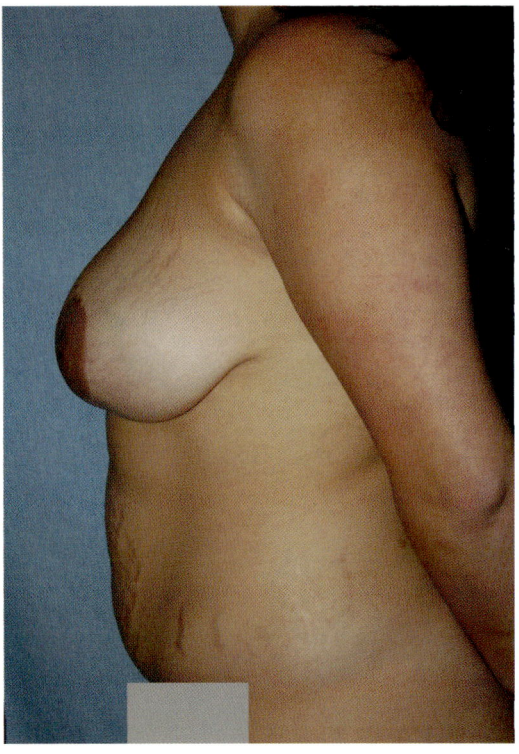 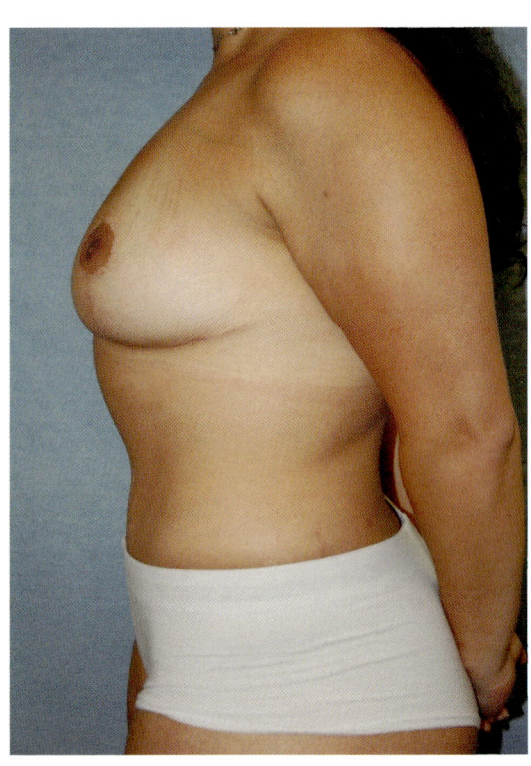

# Breast Lift and Reduction Case 2

Front, angle, and side view

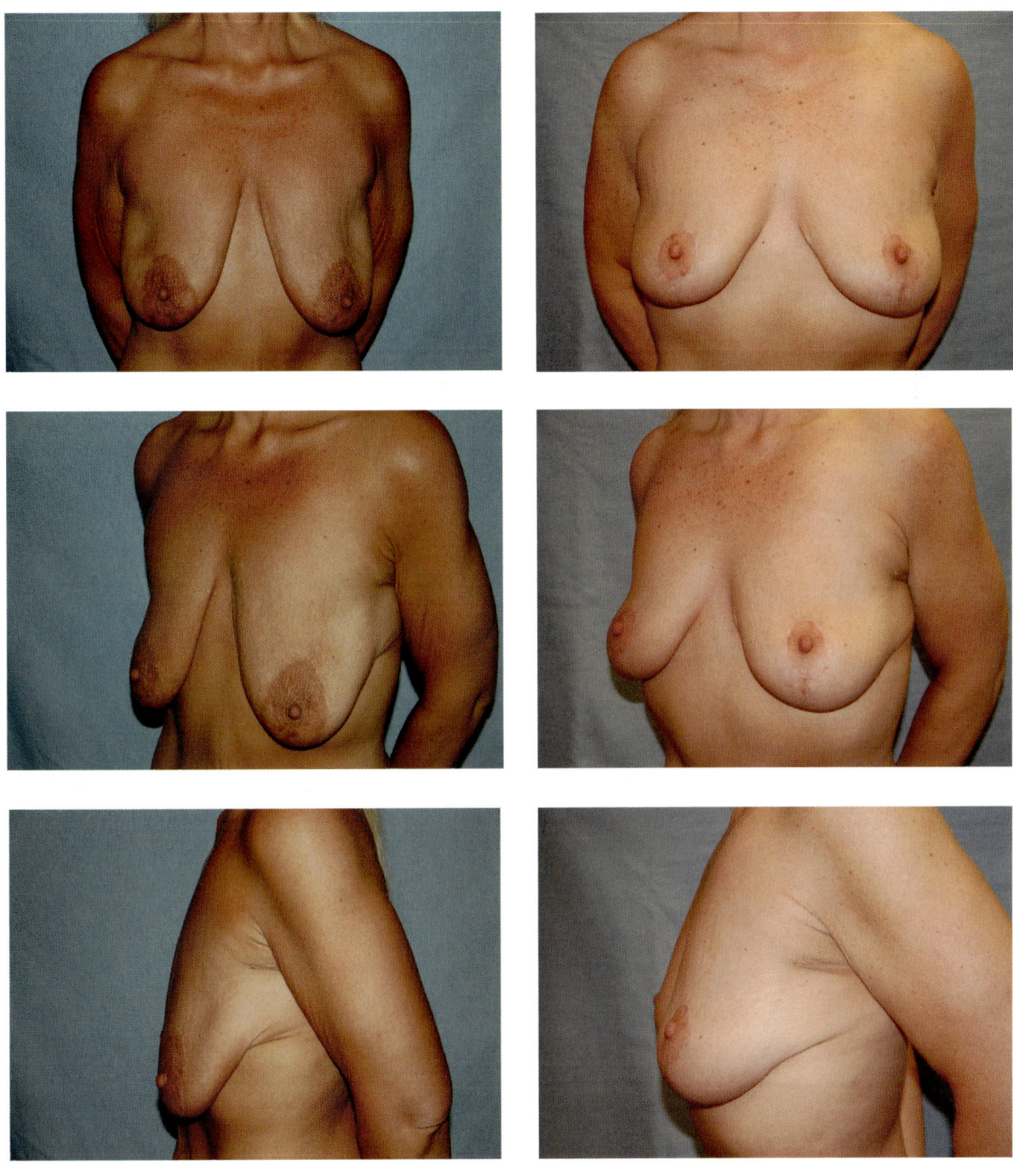

## Breast Lift and Reduction Case 3

Angle
view

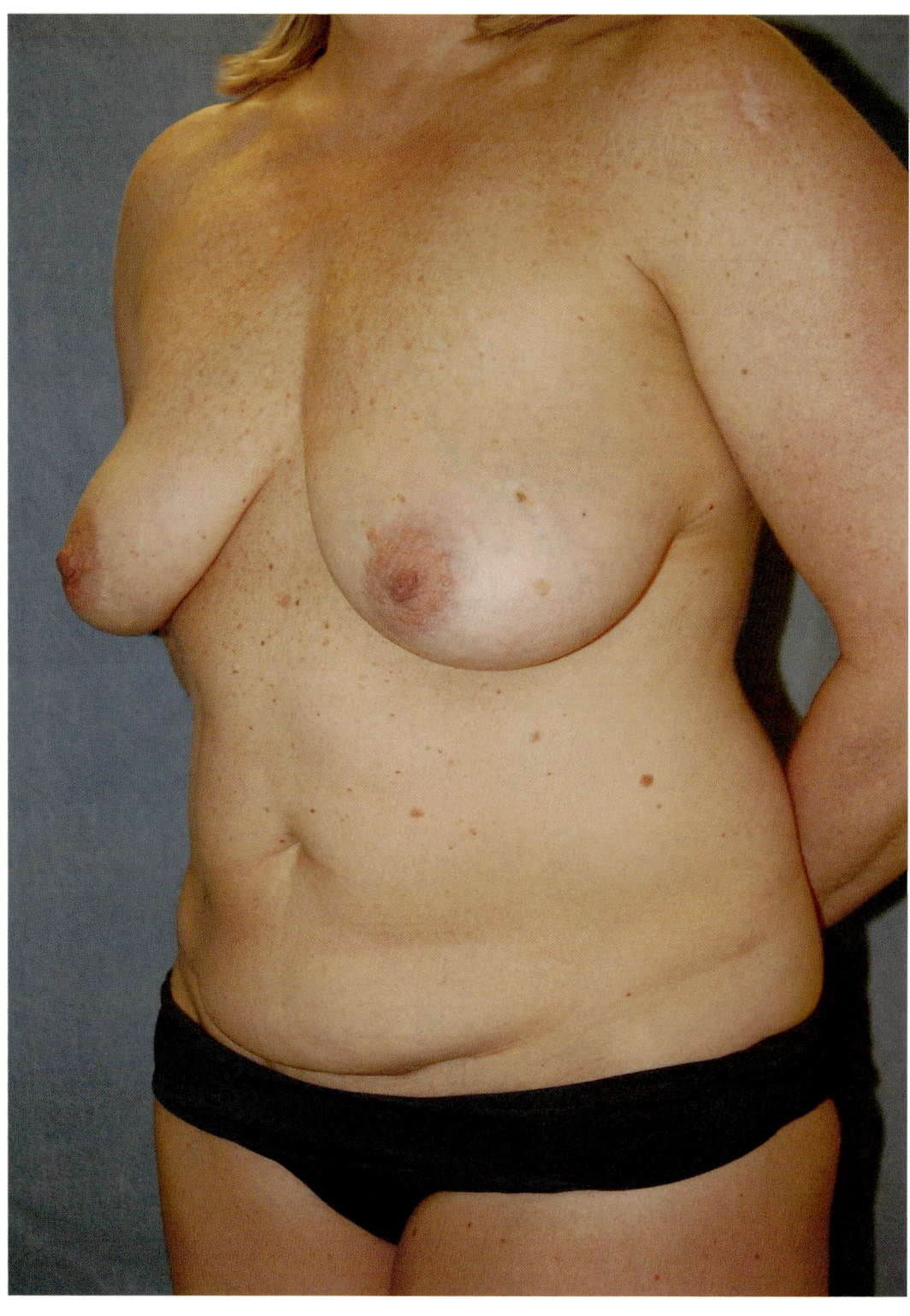

Angle
view

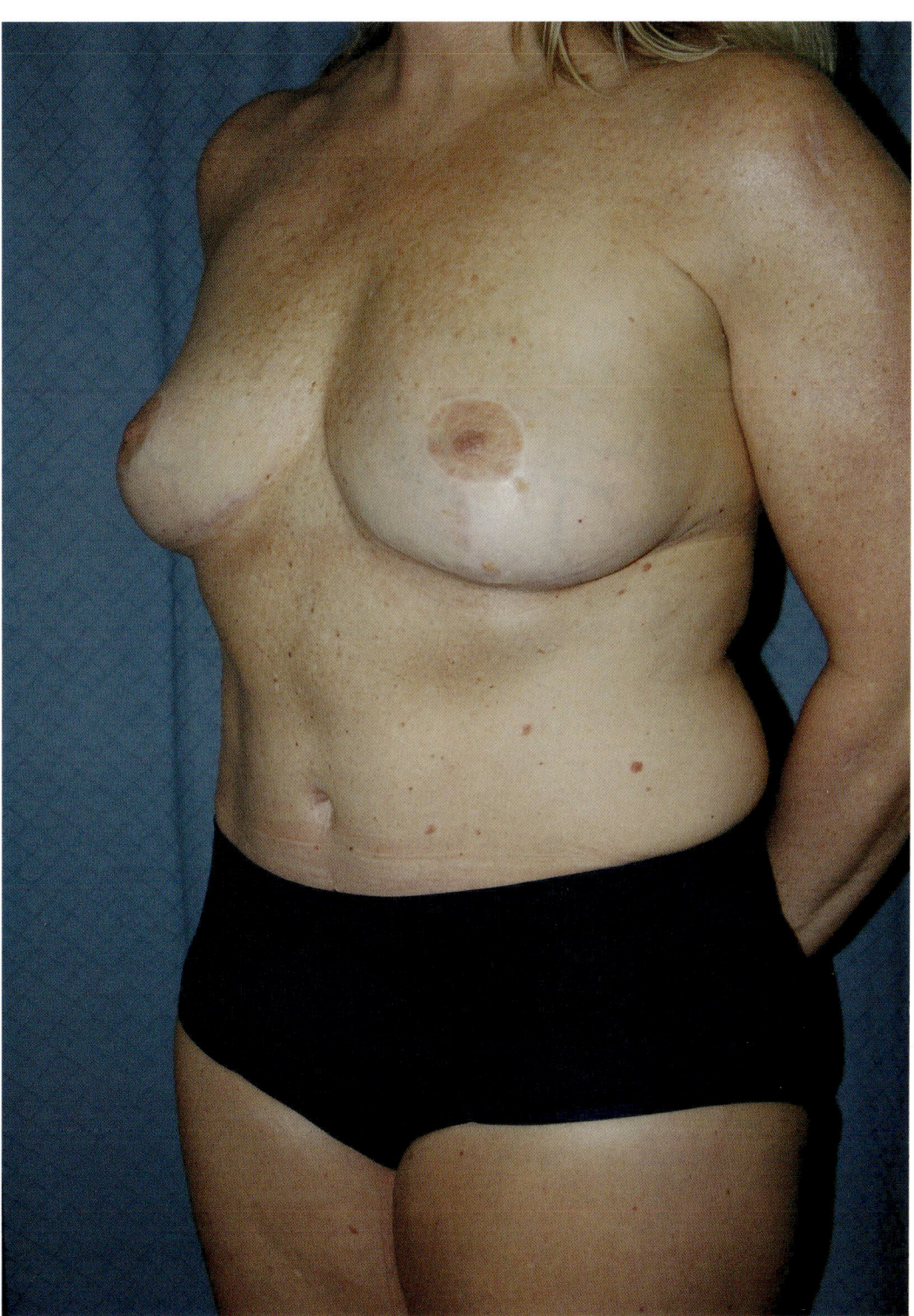

Front view

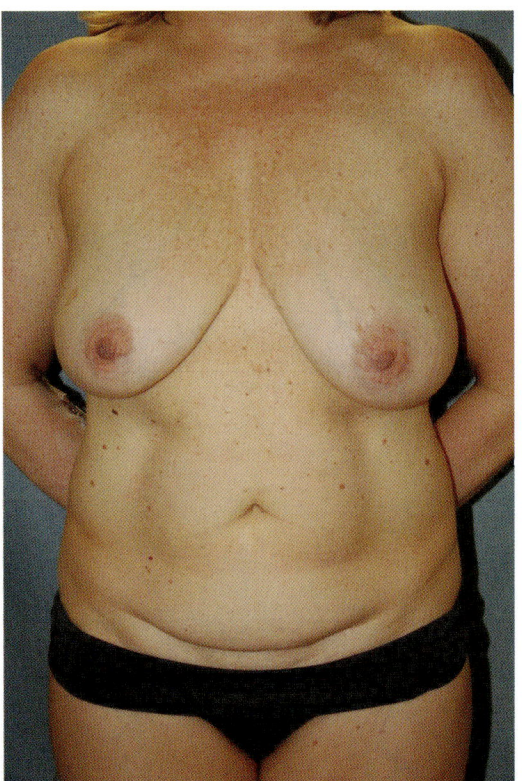 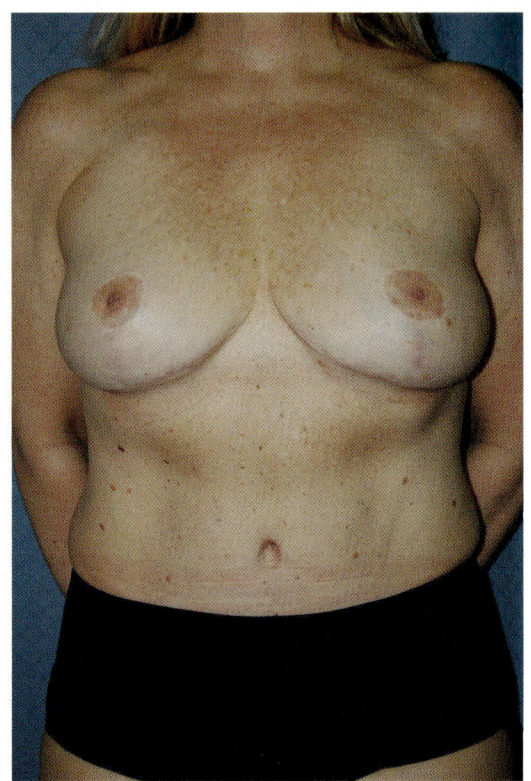

Side view

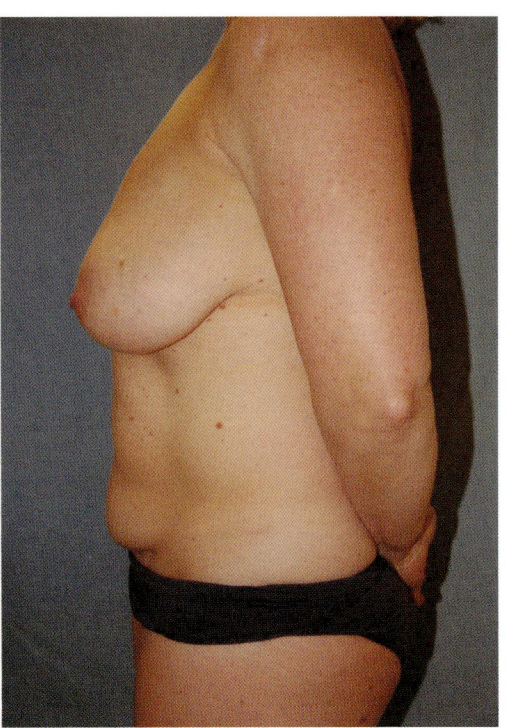 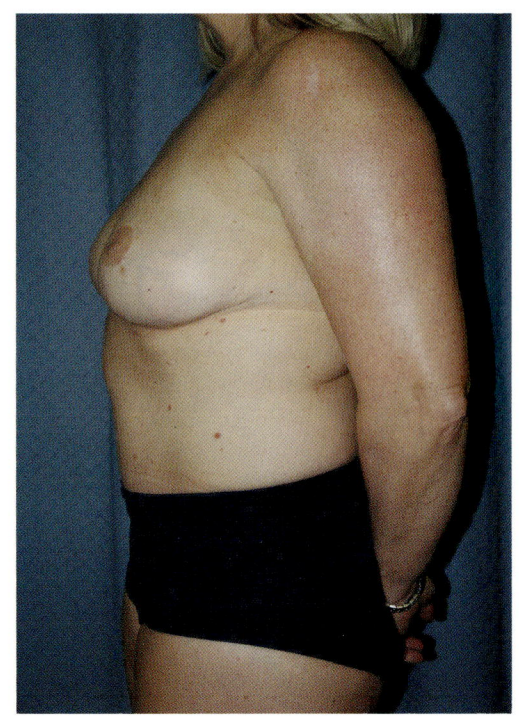

# Lip Filler

Front view

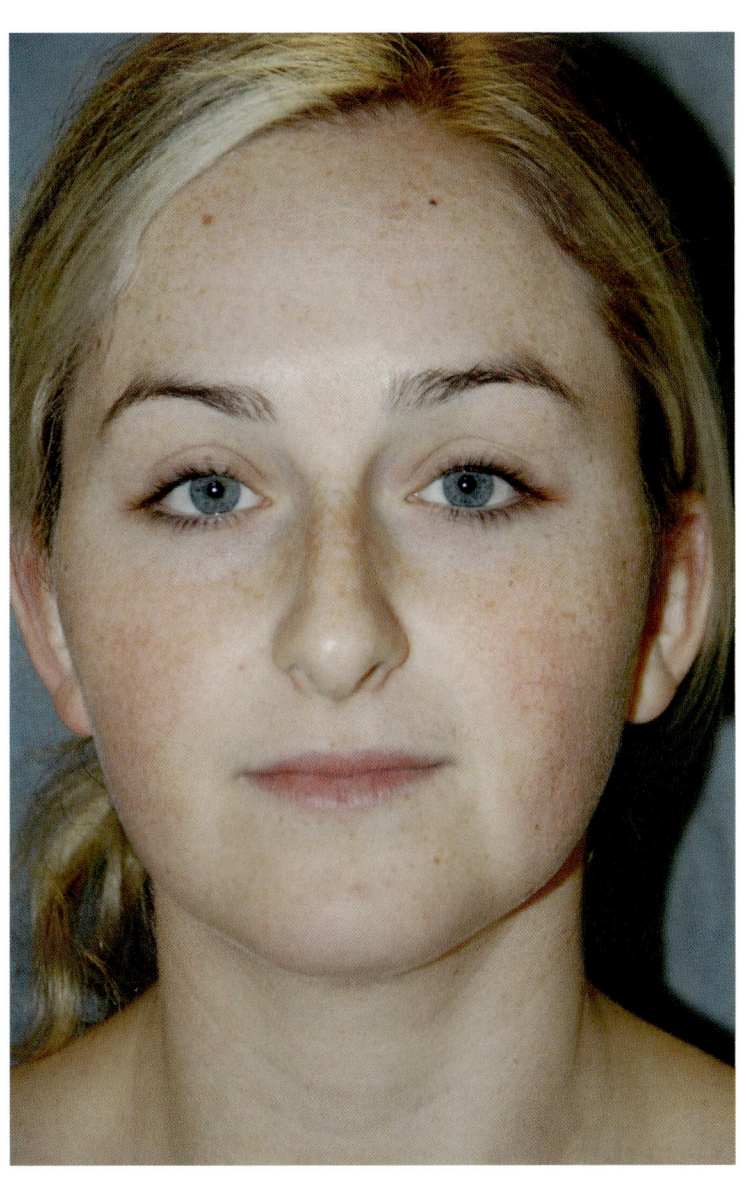
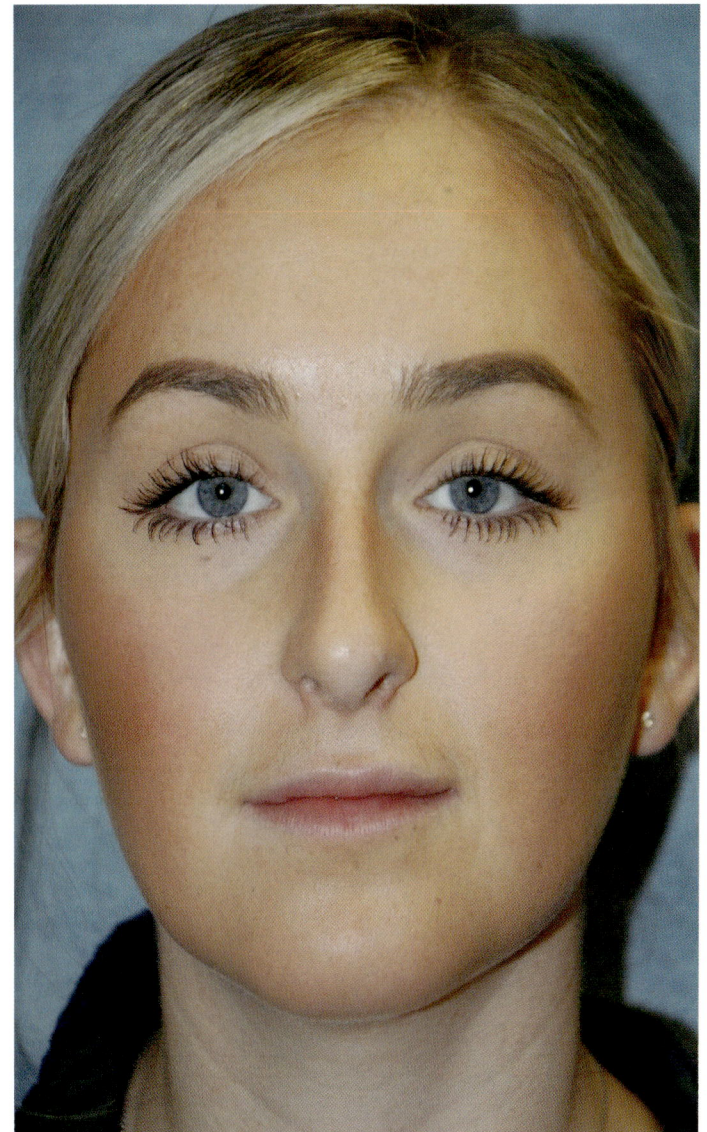

Botox

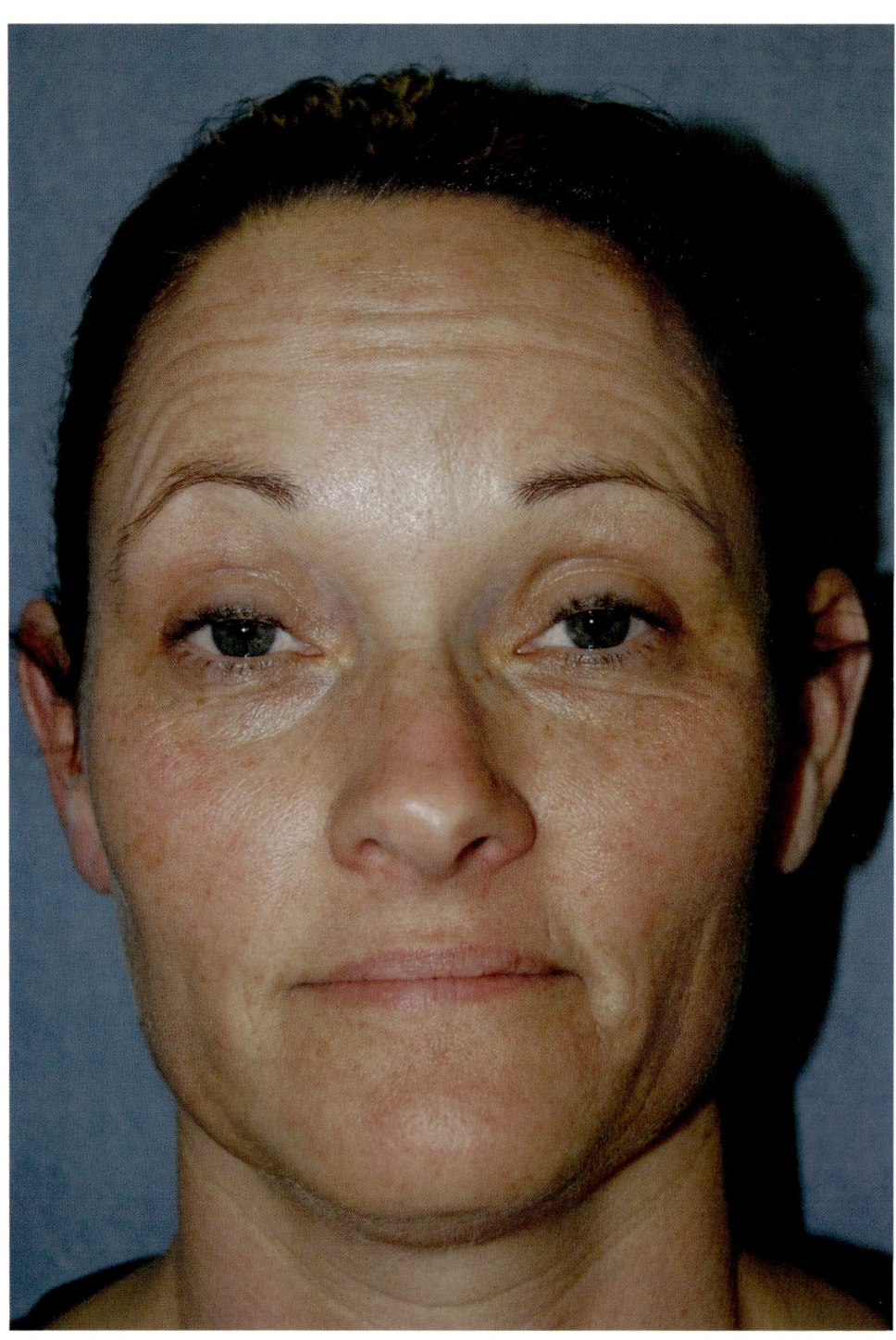

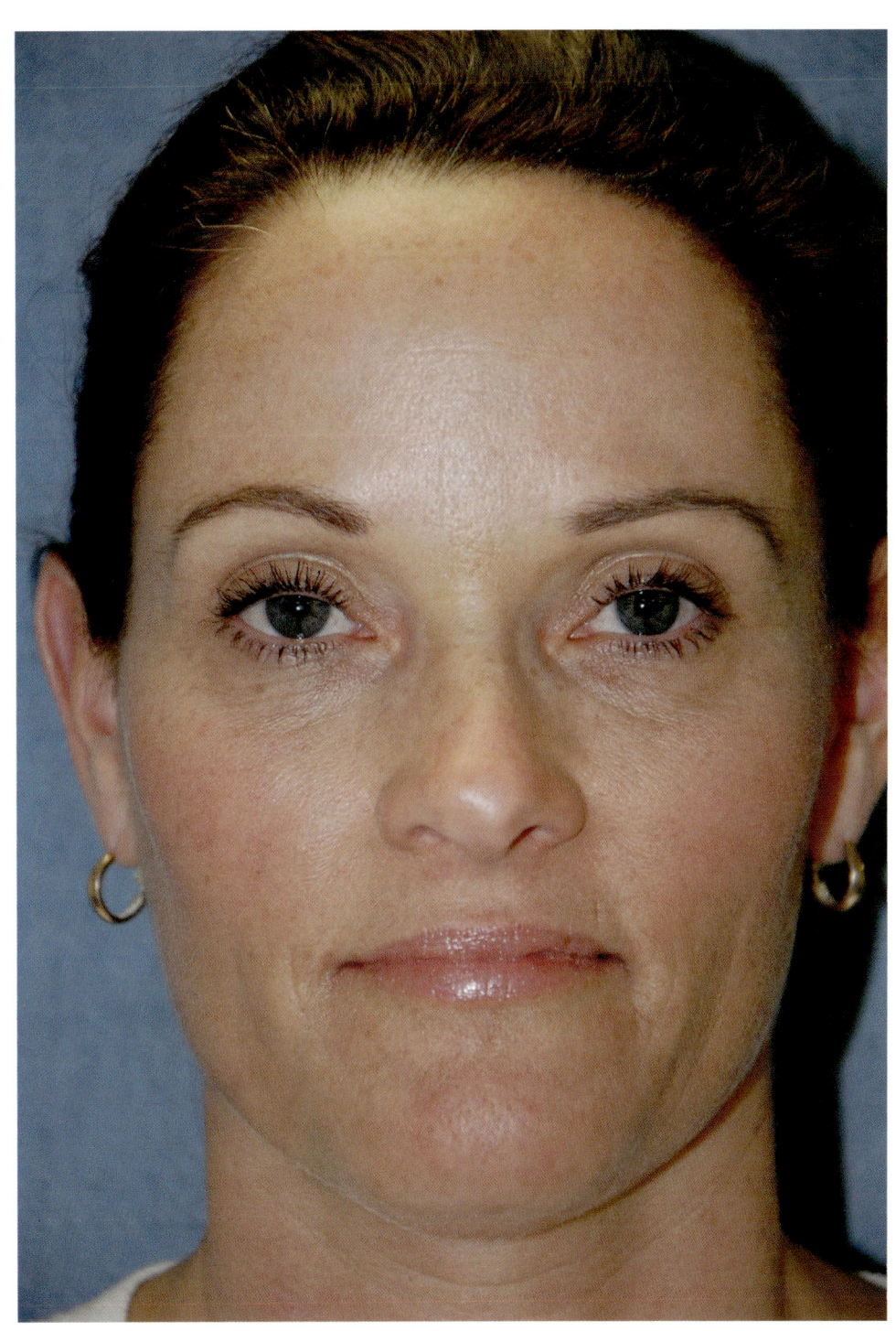